AF271991

1

# Pacemaker Programming – A Handbook

*Eva Clausson*

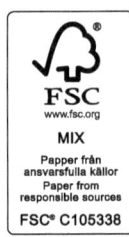

Author: Eva Clausson

Graphic form, illustrations and cover: Eva Clausson, in some cases with permission from Medtronic

Print: BoD

© 2013 Eva Clausson

First edition

ISBN: 9789174633894

# Preface

Ever since the first pacemaker implantation at the Karolinska University hospital in Stockholm, Sweden, on October 8, 1958, much has changed in the field of heart stimulation. The first stimulators were almost the size of a hockey puck and had a battery life limited to a couple of years at most. Now, they are multi-programmable devices that, while weighing only around 30 grams, have hundreds or even thousands of programming combinations, the ability to collect numerous diagnostic data, and longevities that by far exceed those early devices. This development has given us the possibility not only to prolong life, but also to restore quality of life. In the United States, approximately 200 000 new patients have a pacemaker implanted every year, and the number is increasing, both due to the aging population and new indications. Care of these patients includes not only diagnosis and implantation of the pacemaker system but also periodic check-ups of the implanted system using technical measurements and clinically well-grounded programming to assure optimal treatment. For the physicians and nurses caring for and programming these patients, literature describing this process has been scarce. Since the correct programming of the device may very well be the most important aspect of successful treatment, it is my hope that this book will act as a tool for both the beginner and the more experienced caregiver alike, to be read from the beginning to the end or to be used as a reference when questions arise.

*Eva Clausson, August 2013*

# Introduction

## Basic Electrophysiology

Approximately half of human body weight is composed of various kinds of muscle, among which the heart can be seen as the most important. The body consists of three different types of muscle cells: skeletal (controlled by will), smooth (controlled by the autonomic nervous system), and heart muscle cells. Heart and skeletal muscle cells are both striated but have fundamental differences that give the heart muscles their very specialized function. While contraction of the skeletal muscles is initiated by nerve impulses from the brain, the heart muscles have their own control station situated in the right atrium, called the sinus node. The highly specialized cells of the sinus node are connected to the sympathetic and parasympathetic (vagal) nervous system, and they use information from those systems to change the frequency of the heart contractions. This ensures proper blood circulation to meet the ever-varying needs of the body (for example, the need for oxygen). During physical exercise, the pulse frequency from the sinus node increases, leading to more heart contractions per minute and an increased blood flow through the body. The muscle cells of the heart, like the other muscle cells of the body, are activated by small electrical signals that conduct from cell to cell. To maintain a normal heart rhythm, all the components of the heart's electrical system need to work properly.

Some of the heart cells also have the unique ability to start an activation on their own if necessary (for example, if the pulses from the sinus node are absent). This is called automaticity and is available in the electrical conduction system of the heart, where activation is achieved (as in the sinus node) by a slow leakage of ions through the cell membrane, which ultimately leads to self-activation of the cell if not activated by an external signal. This acts as a safety system and may be life-saving in case of failure of the heart's normal electrical system. A slow escape rhythm can thus be maintained, high enough to keep a person alive.

# The Electrical System of the Heart

Thus, the contractions of the heart are controlled by an electrical system consisting of different parts. Assemblages of specialized cells in the right atrium form the *sinus node*. This node receives information from the sympathetic and the parasympathetic nervous system and uses the information to determine what heart rate is needed at any given time. The sinus node then emits small electrical impulses at the right speed, and the heart responds to each signal with a contraction. The propagation of the signal starts in the right atrium and spreads quickly from the sinus node until all muscle cells in the atria have been reached and the atria contract. The atrial muscle cells are connected, allowing the signal to spread from cell to cell, but the valvular plane constitutes an electrically insulated layer that permits the signal to conduct from atria to ventricles. This layer is pierced in only one spot by an electrically conducting structure where the signals are allowed to transfer from atria to ventricles. This thread of cells, named the AV node (atrioventricular node), also causes a delay of the signal on its way down to the ventricles to allow for the atria to contract and empty their blood into the ventricles before ventricular contraction is initiated. The active filling of the ventricles, caused by the atrial contraction, is important to heart function, especially at lower heart rates. When the signal has passed the AV node, it quickly spreads over the ventricles using a specialized conduction system that facilitates a faster conduction than that from cell to cell. The conduction system consists of several bundle branches to quickly reach every part of the ventricles, and by doing so causes an effective contraction of the heart.

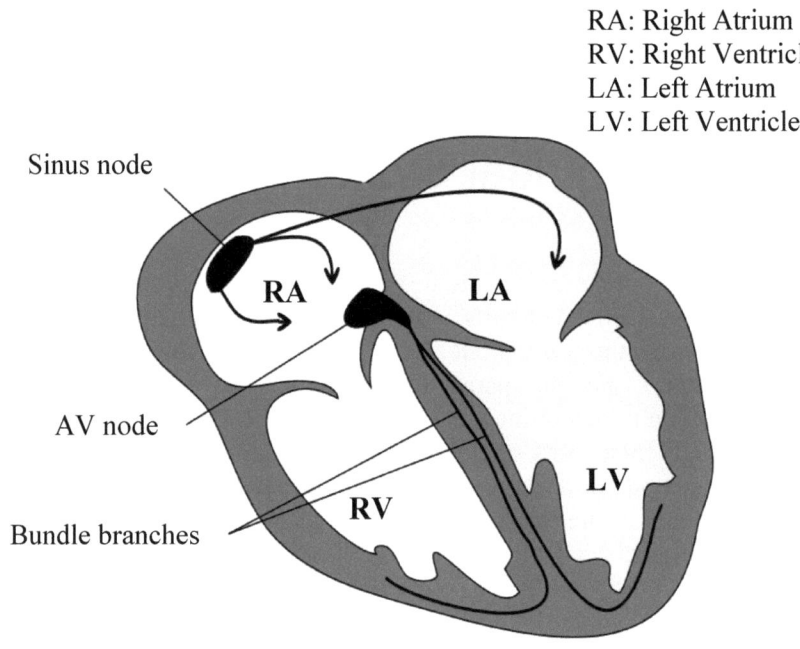

FIGURE 1.1 The electrical system of the heart, consisting of the sinus node (placed in the right atrium), the AV node (piercing the valvular plane in the septum, between atria and ventricles), and the conduction system with bundle braches reaching for the right and left ventricles.

The muscle cells of the heart have a resting potential, measured over the cell membrane, of -90 mV. This difference in potential is caused by an imbalance in the concentration of sodium and potassium ions between the inside and the outside of the cell, created by the sodium-potassium pump. Inside the cell, the concentration of potassium ions is high, while the outside of the cell has a higher concentration of sodium ions. When the cell is stimulated, channels in the cell membrane open up to facilitate an inflow of sodium ions, leading to a changeover in the transmembrane potential from -90 mV to +20-30 mV. The work of the sodium-potassium pump then takes over to restore the potential of -90 mV. This process can be divided into four phases which describe the different states of the cell during activation.

**Depolarization phase:** A fast inflow of sodium ions reverses the transmembrane potential from -90 mV to +20-30 mV.

**Plateau phase:** The permeability of the membrane decreases, and the potential over the cell membrane stabilizes at 0 mV for a short period of time.

**Repolarization phase:** Sodium ions are pumped out from the cell, and the original potential of -90 mV is restored. During this phase the heart cells are in diverging phases of polarization/depolarization, and a new stimuli during this phase may lead to arrhythmia since some cells may be activated and others not. This phase falls into the T wave of the ECG and is commonly referred to as the vulnerable phase. Directly after depolarization (before the vulnerable phase), the heart cells cannot respond to new stimuli. This phase, referred to as the refractory period, lessens the risk for arrhythmias and affects the synchronicity of the heart contraction.

**Resting phase:** The transmembrane potential is back to -90 mV and the cell is ready to be stimulated once more.

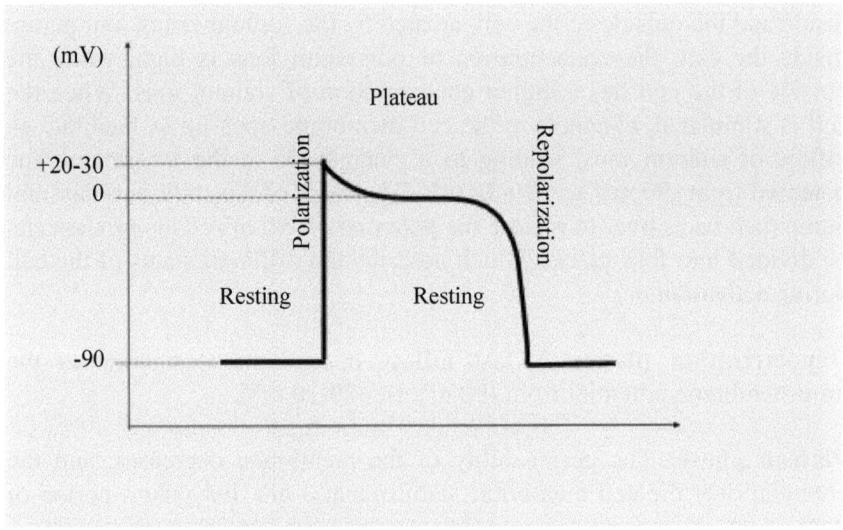

**FIGURE 1.2** The polarization phases of the heart cell

# The ECG

In every heartbeat, all the heart cells are activated in a specific order. The electrical signal from the summed activation of all cells can be visualized by ECG (electrocardiogram), where the respective deflections represent the different activation phases of the atria and the ventricles:

**The P wave:** The depolarization of the atria. The repolarization of the atria cannot be seen on the ECG since it coincides with the depolarization of the ventricles and thus hides within that larger signal.

**The QRS complex:** The depolarization of the ventricles.

**The T wave:** The repolarization of the ventricles.

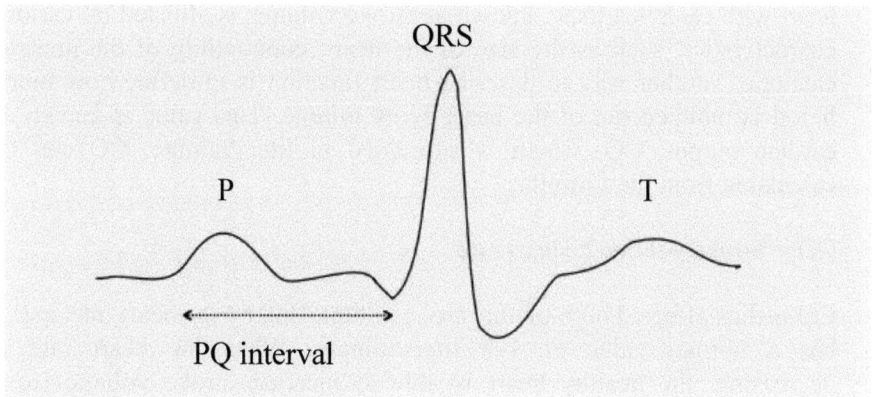

**FIGURE 1.3** ECG with the respective reflections marked out. The P wave represents the atrial depolarization. The interval between the P wave and the QRS complex (the depolarization of the ventricles) represents the delay of the signal in the AV node, named PQ interval. Finally, the T wave represents the repolarization of the ventricles.

# Stroke Volume and Cardiac Output

The heart's ability to provide the body with blood is dependent upon many different factors. The amount of blood that is pumped out of the heart with each heartbeat, known as stroke volume, is affected by various characterstics, such as the size of the heart, contractility of the muscle, etcetera. Another way to describe heart function is to define how much blood is pumped out of the heart every minute. This value is known as cardiac output, CO, which is expressed in liters/minute. CO can be calculated from the formula:

CO = Stroke volume * Heart rate

CO is thus affected both by the stroke volume and by the heart rate, and it has a normal value of 4–8 liters/minute. When the heart rate is decreasing, the healthy heart is able to increase stroke volume (to a certain limit) to compensate, but if the heart rate becomes too slow, CO will become too low to satisfy the body's needs (for example, oxygen). This may lead to symptoms such as fatigue, dizziness and syncope.

# Bradycardia

Heart rates below 40 beats/minute, commonly known as bradycardia, may originate from different parts of the heart's electrical system. The two most common reasons for slow heart rate are sinus node dysfunction and electrical block between the atria and ventricles in the AV node (AV block). Patients with symptomatic bradycardia are commonly treated with implantation of a pacemaker. The pacemaker then either simulates the function of the sinus node and sends out small electrical pulses to control the heart rhythm or substitutes the AV node function by conducting the electrical signals from atria to ventricles.

Bradyarrhythmias may affect individuals of all ages, and pacemaker treatment may be indicated for a small child as well as for a 100-year-old. Most commonly, however, symptomatic bradycardia debuts after the age of 70, and the mean age for the first implantation is around 75 years. The most common indications for pacing are:

- Sick sinus syndrome
- AV block I
- AV block II type 1 (Wenckebach)
- AV block II type 2 (2:1 or higher)
- AV block III
- Atrial fibrillation with slow ventricular response

## AV Block

The most common indication for pacing is AV block (AVB) of different degrees. These may be of a chronic or intermittent nature. The degree of AVB is defined by the function of the AV node, where AVB I means a prolongation in the conduction time from atria to ventricles (prolonged PQ interval). AVB I is usually defined as conduction times >200 ms (>220 ms for patients older than 60 years). In AVB II, some of the signals from the atria are conducted to the ventricles while others are blocked. The pattern by which conduction occurs defines the type of AVB II, for example Wenckebach (AVB II type 1) or 2:1 block (AVB II type 2).

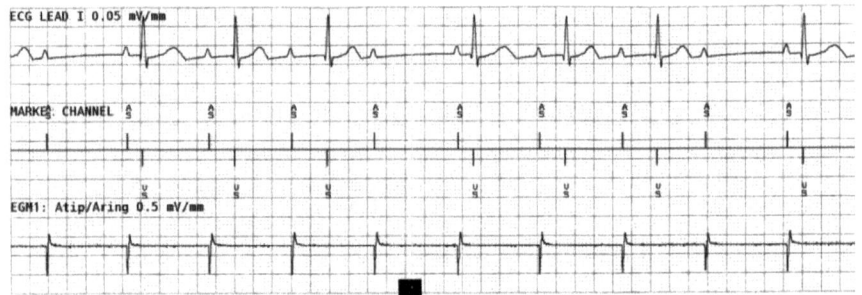

**FIGURE 1.4** AVB II type 1, Wenckebach block. Note the increased PQ interval that finally leads to one blocked P wave, after which the sequence is repeated

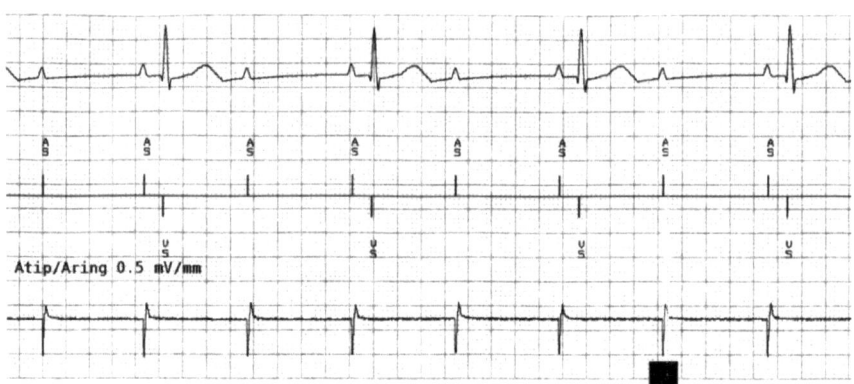

**FIGURE 1.5** AVB II type 2, 2:1-block. Only every second P wave is conducted to the ventricles leading to a QRS complex

In AVB III, all P waves are blocked on their way to the ventricles. When this happens, a slow ventricular rhythm may be triggered by the ventricular conduction system. The resulting rate is commonly no more than 30 min$^{-1}$, which may trigger symptoms such as lightheadedness,

18

presyncope or syncope. It is not uncommon that the bradycardia is preceded by a short asystole, which may in itself cause syncope.

## Sick Sinus Syndrome

Sick sinus syndrome is a generic name for a variety of syndromes initiated in the sinus node that lead to an inadequately low heart rate. This may manifest itself as bradycardia, sinus arrests or inability to adequately increase heart rate during exercise (chronotropic incompetence). Patients with sick sinus syndrome also have a much higher prevalence of atrial fibrillation than the rest of the population. With pacemaker treatment, we aim at maintaining adequate heart rate during sinus bradycardia and also stabilizing and increasing the heart rate for patients with atrial fibrillation and a slow ventricular response. There is some clinical evidence that a programmed lower rate of 70 min$^{-1}$ may have a preventive effect on the number of AF attacks[1].

# Different Pacemaker Systems

Choosing a pacemaker system is dependent upon the indication for pacing for the individual patient. We need to take into account the acute needs as well as possible future needs if the disease progresses. Additionally, it is not uncommon that incomplete information is known about the electrical status of the patient's heart before implant. There may be an ECG showing intermittent AV block, but information about chronotropic competence may be lacking. The modern pacemaker contains many functions that can be switched on or off when necessary, but it is nevertheless important to ensure that the proposed system can also provide the functions the patient may need in the upcoming years.

Pacemaker treatment should always aim at restoring normal heart rhythm, meaning that the device should only take over functions that are not working properly. The chosen pacemaker system should therefore neither result in over- nor under-treatment. Pacemaker systems are commonly divided into two groups: single-chamber and dual-chamber devices. These differ from each other in the number of leads placed in the heart. The single-chamber system is connected to one lead placed in the atrium or in the ventricle, while the dual chamber system is connected to two leads, one in the atrium *and* one in the ventricle. The indications for pacing determine which system should be used.

## The Single-Chamber System

A single-chamber pacemaker system consists of the pulse generator (pacemaker) connected to a lead (cable) placed either in the right atrium or the right ventricle. Systems using a lead only in the atrium require an intact conduction from atrium to ventricle (fully functioning AV node) and may be used in sinus node disease without AV block. However, this is an uncommon therapy today due to reasons discussed later in this book.

Single-chamber systems with the lead placed in the right ventricle are used in patients with permanent atrial fibrillation (since it is then not possible to stimulate or to use the atria for deciding heart rate) and in patients with a sporadic need for pacing where the device is only used as protection against syncope. Even so, it is always important to take into account that the need for pacing may increase over time and that the patient may then need an upgrade to a dual-chamber system.

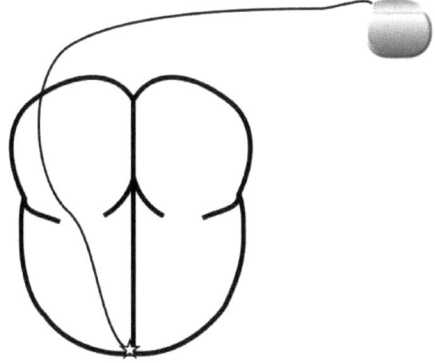

FIGURE 1.6 The single-chamber system with one lead, here placed in the right ventricle

## The Dual-Chamber System

A dual-chamber system consists of the pulse generator connected to two leads. One of the leads is placed in the right atrium (most commonly in the right atrial appendix), and the other is placed in the right ventricle (most commonly in the ventricular apex). The dual-chamber system can be seen as a universal system that can be used to treat sick sinus syndrome as well as AV block. In sick sinus syndrome, the atria are stimulated in the same way as with the single-chamber system, with a lead in the atrium. The ventricular lead is then used as a backup if AV block should develop.

In AV block, the atrial lead is used to sense the activity in the atria, which the pacemaker helps by conducting to the ventricles via the ventricular lead. In this way a physiologic activation of the heart can be achieved, with the atria and ventricles in sequence, and a natural rate adaption can be provided by the sinus node.

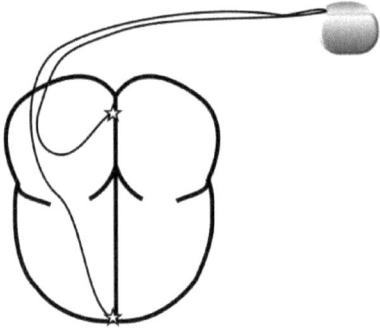

**FIGURE 1.7** The dual-chamber system with one lead placed in the right atrium and one lead in the right ventricle

# Why Do We Program?

As previously mentioned in the preface, the indication for a modern pacemaker is not simply to provide life-supporting therapy; in some cases, it may just serve as a tool to increase quality of life. Guidelines recommend that a pacemaker be implanted when the patient shows symptoms of bradycardia, and a sole finding of slow heart rate on ECG is thus not reason enough. However, it is not always easy to determine whether symptoms are present or not, since average age for a patient at the first implantation is around 75 years of age (and some patients are significantly older). As well, symptoms of bradycardia such as exercise intolerance, shortness of breath, dizziness and syncope are common in this age group and may be overlooked as normal (both by the patient and the physician). It is not rare to meet with patients at the first follow-up after implantation and hear them say that they feel at least ten years younger! To achieve the best possible results from the treatment, it is very important that the pacemaker is correctly programmed for the individual patient, which includes a whole range of parameters. The given indications affect both which system to choose and how that system should be programmed to best suit the patient's needs. Every patient is unique with regard to pacemaker programming, and it should be the natural right for each patient to have his or her pacemaker correctly programmed for their needs. It can directly affect the patient's perception of well-being, and in some cases may even determine whether the patient later develops atrial fibrillation or even heart failure.

# The NBG Code

To simplify the way we quote the basic function of the pacemaker, we are using the so-called NBG code. Since a modern pacemaker is not only delivering electrical pulses but also has the ability to sense the intrinsic heartbeats, it can adapt its way of working, beat by beat, to the patient's intrinsic heart rhythm. The NBG code is an international code system that describes the basic function of the pacemaker using both where stimulation and sensing takes place as well as its basic way of working. NBG is short for NASPE/BPEG generic pacemaker code and is thus the result of cooperation between the North American (NASPE, North American Society of Pacing and Electrophysiology) and the British (BPEG, British Pacing & Electrophysiology Group) societies of pacing and electrophysiology. The code is built upon three- or four-letter combinations, where each position (I-IV) has a specific meaning.

**Position I:** The first position states in which chamber/chambers of the heart the device is stimulating. This can be in the atrium (A), the ventricle (V), both chambers (D=Dual), or not at all (O).

**Position II:** The second position states in which chamber/chambers of the heart the device is sensing. This can also be in the atrium (A), the ventricle (V), both chambers (D=Dual), or not at all (O).

**Position III:** The third position states the reaction of the device when sensing occurs. The reaction may be inhibition (I), meaning that after sensing of an intrinsic heartbeat, the next planned stimulation pulse in this heart chamber will be withheld (inhibited). This is the most common function in single-chamber pacemakers (AAI, VVI).

When using a pacemaker to overcome AV block, the activity of the sinus node is sensed by the atrial lead, and every sensed signal initiates an AV interval. If the AV interval is allowed to expire (meaning that no ventricular signal is sensed), a pulse is delivered in the ventricle. This behavior is called tracking. Thus, the dual-chamber pacemaker also has a dual function (D) in that it inhibits stimulation pulses in the chamber where sensing occurred (I) and also facilitates ventricular pacing after atrial sensing.

The first pacemakers developed were of the type VOO, lacking sensing capabilities, and they thereby paced at a fixed rate. This could lead to problems from time to time when stimulation in the vulnerable phase of the T wave resulted in arrhythmias. To avoid this, it was necessary to develop a pacemaker that took into account the spontaneous rhythm of the heart, but since the technology at that point in time did not provide electronic counters like the ones we use today, it was not possible to inhibit the pacing pulses. Instead, the solution came in a system that also delivered a pulse every time it sensed intrinsic activity. In this way pulses could be synchronized to the R wave, eliminating the risks associated with pacing in the vulnerable phase. However, these systems were wasting energy since every heart cycle by default had to include a stimulation pulse, even when it was not clinically indicated. The letter T stands for this triggered behavior.

An "O" in the third position means "no function" and will always be the case when the letter O is found in position II. If there is no sensing, there cannot be a reaction to sensing.

**Position IV:** In this position we find codes which some use to describe older pacemaker functions. The first pacemaker models manufactured were neither programmable nor equipped with telemetry to retrieve saved data, such as the models of today. An "O" in the fourth position stands for the way these early devices functioned. When technology improved, it was possible to develop devices with limited programming capabilities, such as programmable rate and pulse amplitude. This behavior is indicated by the letter "P" (Programmable). The next step was multi-programmable devices (M), and after that came devices with telemetry to read stored data from the device (C=Communication). When looking at the devices of today, all of them are probably both multi-programmable and equipped with telemetry, and at the same time include a function called rate response (R), which means they incorporate one or more sensors to increase the heart rate when needed (for example if the patient is physically active). An "R" in the fourth position means that the pacemaker is multi-programmable, has telemetry and includes rate response.

| Position | I | II | III | IV |
|---|---|---|---|---|
| | Chamber paced | Chamber sensed | Reaction to sensing | Programmability |
| | O = None | O = None | O = None | O = None |
| | A = Atrium | A = Atrium | T = Triggered | P = Programmable |
| | V = Ventricle | V = Ventricle | I = Inhibited | M = Multi programmable |
| | D = Dual (A+V) | D = Dual (A+V) | D = Dual (T+I) | C = Communication |
| Manufacturer's denotation | S = Single (A or V) | S = Single (A or V) | | R = Rate response |

Table 3.1 The letter combinations of the NBG code

26

# Basic Parameters

## Mode

Mode is the most fundamental pacemaker parameter and can be directly derived from the NBG code in the chapter above. The decision of mode naturally follows the choice of a system that optimally meets the needs of the patient. The system should meet present needs as well as possible future changes in that need. Should the patient receive a single- or dual-chamber device? If a single-chamber device is chosen, a decision needs to be made whether to implant the lead in the atrium (AAI) or in the ventricle (VVI). After this decision, the conditions for programming are set. For the single-chamber device, the modes VVI/R and AAI/R are exclusively used. For dual-chamber devices, DDD/R is most commonly used, but devices are occasionally permanently programmed to DDI/R. Beyond this, there are numerous other modes available which are seldom or never used permanently. For example, AOO, VOO and DOO are used when fixed stimulation is delivered on the implanted lead/leads, and OAO, OVO or ODO are used when the pacemaker is switched off.

### AAI

An AAI pacemaker is connected to one lead that stimulates and senses the right atrium. The pacemaker is active when the intrinsic rate falls below the programmed lower rate, and stimulation is given at the lower rate. In the case of intrinsic atrial rates above lower rate, stimulation is inhibited and the pacemaker is passive. AAI is the mode least used among the ones described here. Patients with sick sinus syndrome may be indicated for an AAI system (preferably with a rate response function, AAIR), but in clinical praxis these patients are more often fitted with a DDDR system. This choice is due to the somewhat increased prevalence of AV block in this patient population as well as an increased risk for developing atrial fibrillation.

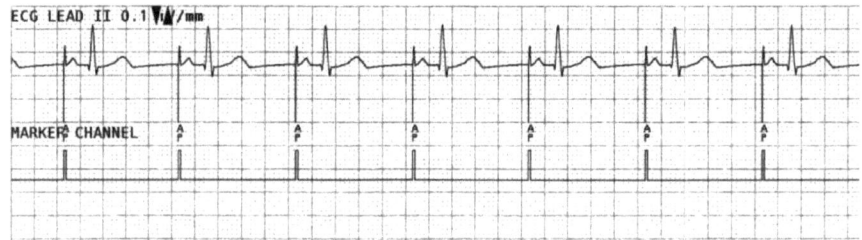

FIGURE 4.1 Example of an ECG during AAI mode

# VVI

A VVI pacemaker is connected to one lead that stimulates and senses the right ventricle. The pacemaker is active when the intrinsic ventricular rate falls below the programmed lower rate, and stimulation is given at the lower rate. In the case of intrinsic ventricular rates above lower rate, stimulation is inhibited and the pacemaker is passive. Patients with permanent atrial fibrillation in conjunction with bradycardia are indicated for a VVIR system, since the atria cannot be used as a natural pacemaker or be stimulated during atrial fibrillation. In rare cases, patients with little stimulation need are fitted with a VVI/R system to protect against syncope. However, it is important to remember that the need for stimulation often increases over time and that the VVI/R system may then need to be upgraded with an atrial lead to a DDDR system.

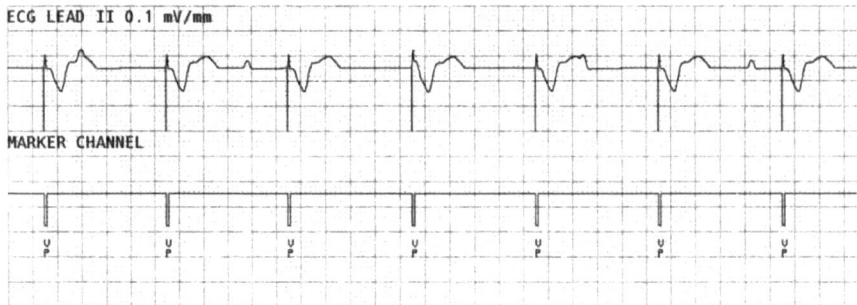

**FIGURE 4.2** Example of an ECG during VVI mode

# DDD

A DDD pacemaker (also called a dual-chamber system) is connected to two leads, one stimulating and sensing the right atrium and one stimulating and sensing the right ventricle. Atrial stimulation starts when the intrinsic atrial rate falls below the lower rate, and stimulation is given at lower rate. Ventricular stimulation follows stimulated or sensed atrial events, after the programmed AV Interval (so-called tracking). Inhibition of atrial stimulation occurs after atrial sensing, and inhibition of ventricular stimulation occurs after ventricular sensing. DDD mode, with or without addition of rate response (DDDR), can be used for most pacemaker indications: sick sinus syndrome, AV block, and paroxysmal atrial fibrillation with slow ventricular response (all but permanent atrial fibrillation or flutter). Special attention is necessary when programming the other parameters in order to further adapt the system to the indication and to the individual needs.

29

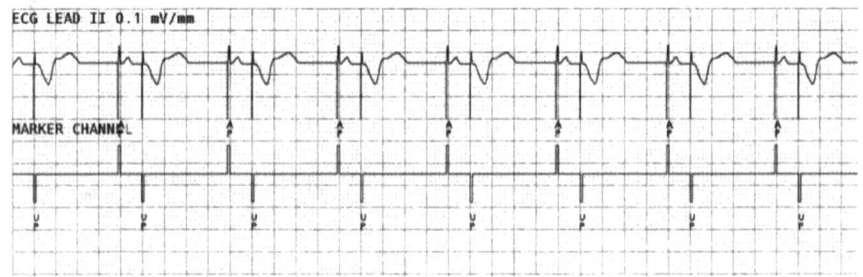

**FIGURE 4.3** Example of an ECG during DDD mode

# DDI

DDI mode was first developed to prevent the pacemaker from tracking fast atrial arrhythmias down to the ventricles (for example, during atrial fibrillation), a problem existing in DDD mode. We don't refer to devices as DDI pacemakers, since DDI is just one of the modes available in a DDD pacemaker. In DDI mode, both atrium and ventricle are stimulated as well as sensed. Inhibition occurs after sensing, but unlike the DDD mode there is *no* tracking available, meaning that a sensed atrial event will *not* start an AV Interval. However, a stimulation pulse in the atrium will start an AV interval, and during atrial stimulation the atria and the ventricles will be synchronized. DDI mode can be seen as an AAI mode with a VVI backup, and it should be avoided during AV block. An undesired behavior in DDI mode during AV block is that an atrial rhythm, if faster than the lower rate, will inhibit atrial stimulation while the ventricles are stimulated at the lower rate. The ECG will then be equivalent to VVI mode, and the patient may experience pacemaker syndrome caused by the atria contracting against closed heart valves. This behavior can be very symptomatic in some patients, and to prevent this from happening, DDI mode is commonly combined with rate response,

30

DDIR, which is also the mode used in most pacemakers when mode-switching during atrial arrhythmias occurs. In DDIR, a higher percentage of atrial pacing can be achieved, leading to better AV synchronization.

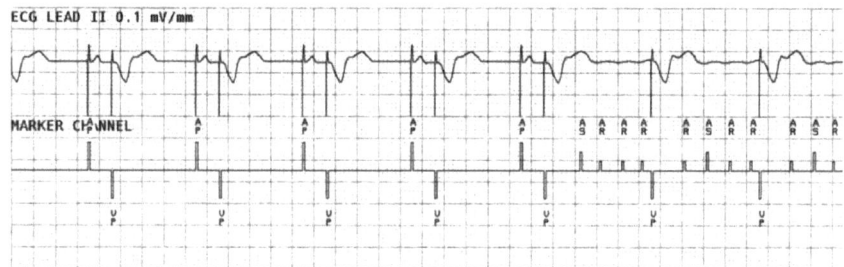

**FIGURE 4.4** Example of an ECG during DDI mode. Synchronized stimulation can be seen in the beginning of the tracing, which toward the end changes to ventricular pacing only, when atrial fibrillation is initiated.

# Amplitude and Pulse Width

The pacemaker delivers electrical pulses to the heart via the leads, and it is of highest importance that all pulses delivered initiate a contraction. When a pulse leads to contraction, it is referred to as capture. Inversely, a pulse that does not succeed in capturing the heart and causing a contraction is referred to as exit block. The amount of energy delivered to the heart by the pulse determines whether capture will be achieved or not, and it is programmed by the parameters of amplitude and pulse width. The amplitude is the strength of the pulse, while the pulse width is the time during which the pulse is delivered. Together with the impedance in the electrical circuit, these two parameters define the energy delivered.

31

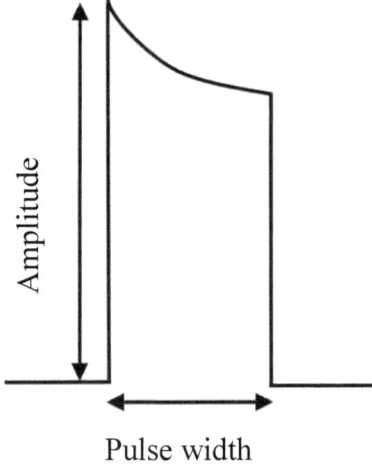

Pulse width

**FIGURE 4.5** The pacemaker pulse

## Stimulation Threshold and the Strength-Duration Curve

The energy needed to capture the heart is dependent upon several factors and differs between patients, between stimulation sites in the same patient, and with different lead types, etc. To define the relationship between capture and the energy delivered by the pacemaker, the strength-duration curve is used. This curve differs between patients but always follows the same algorithm. For all combinations of amplitude and pulse width falling below the curve, there will be no capture, while all combinations that are found above the curve will result in capture (contraction of the heart). The curve itself represents the threshold value for stimulation, meaning the lowest amount of energy needed to capture the heart. Every coordinate on the curve gives a combination of amplitude and pulse width which will result in an energy corresponding to the threshold value. Note that the amount of energy includes both a value for amplitude and for pulse width. The threshold value may and, as an example, be described as 0.5 V@0.4 ms.

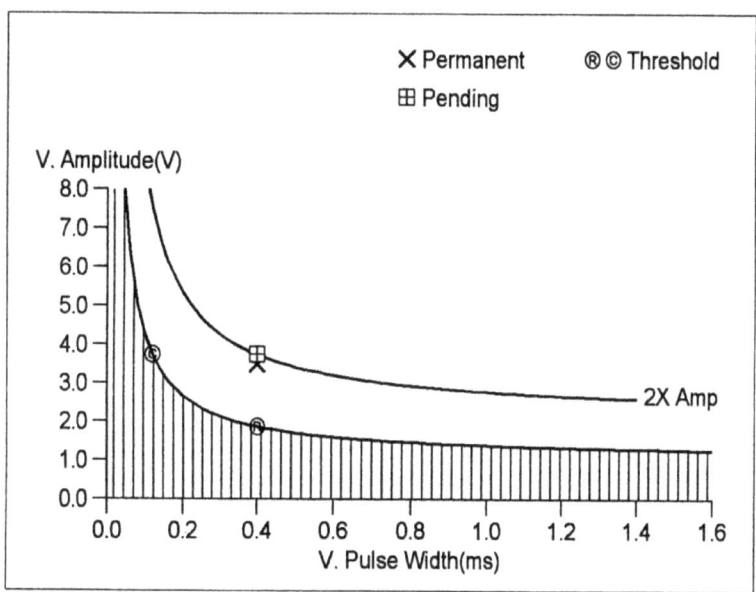

**FIGURE 4.6** The strength-duration curve

The only time we may influence the threshold value is at implantation. Once the lead is in place, a threshold measurement is taken and if the resulting value is not satisfactory (target value below approximately 1 V@0.4 ms), the lead is usually repositioned until a site with acceptable measured values is found.

33

Threshold measurement can be performed in two different ways. The goal is to define a coordinate on the strength-duration curve that may be used as a reference when choosing amplitude/pulse width. The approach is the same whether the measurement is taken during implantation or with a pacemaker programmer during follow-up. The measurement starts at a stimulation amplitude/pulse width large enough to cause capture. The amplitude or the pulse width is then decreased until loss of capture is noted on surface ECG. The lowest value resulting in capture is noted as the threshold value.

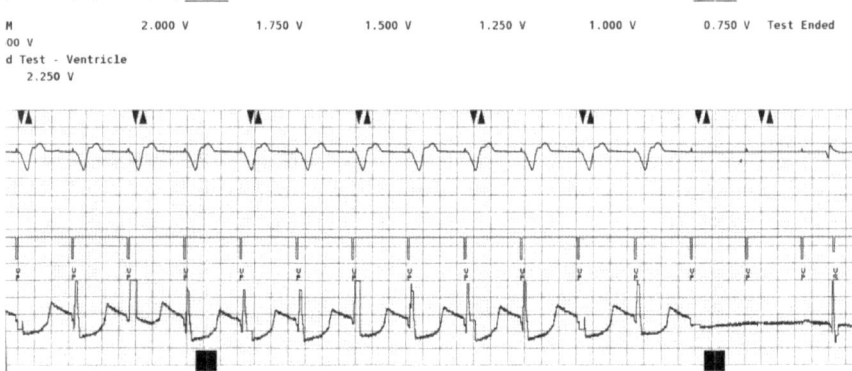

**FIGURE 4.7** Threshold test performed in VVI by decreasing the pulse amplitude. 1.0 V does not result in capture, the threshold is noted to 1.25 V@0.4 ms.

## Measuring Atrial Threshold

When measuring atrial threshold, it is not uncommon to have difficulties seeing the P wave resulting from the stimulation pulse. When this is the case, two tricks may be useful in finding the correct threshold value. Which trick to use depends on the patient's intrinsic rhythm. When intrinsic AV conduction is present, the pacemaker may be programmed in such a way that the intrinsic ventricular complexes are promoted. This is done by temporarily programming the mode to either AAI or DDD with an extended AV interval. Each atrial pulse with capture will now lead to a spontaneous *ventricular* complex, which is used to judge whether atrial capture is present or not. For patients with AV block and intrinsic sinus rhythm, the sensed P waves will return when the atrial pulses no longer have capture. This is commonly seen on the marker channel as refractory senses (AR). When these are noted, it is very likely that the threshold value has been passed.

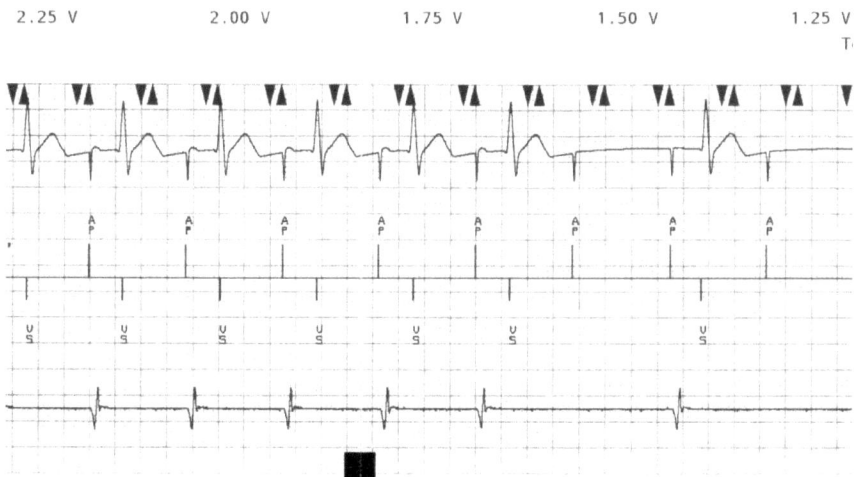

FIGURE 4.8 Atrial threshold test in AAI mode in a patient without AV block. Note the loss of *R wave* when atrial capture is no longer maintained.

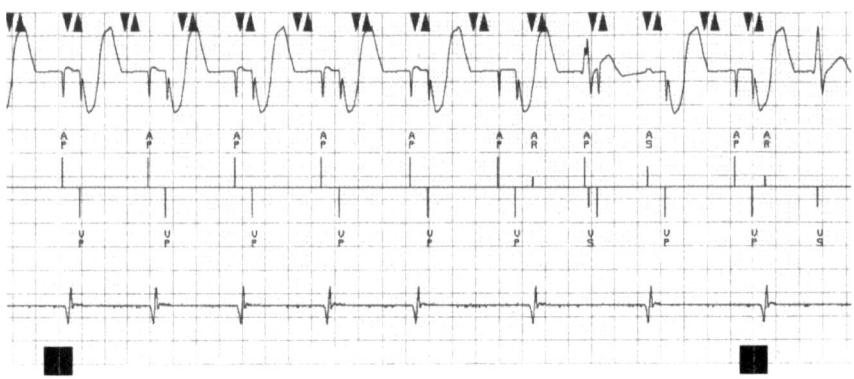

2.25 V          2.00 V          1.75 V          1.50 V     1.25 V     Test Ended

**FIGURE 4.9** Atrial threshold test in DDD in a patient with AV block and intrinsic sinus rhythm. Note the appearance of intrinsic atrial signals (AR) when capture is no longer maintained and the sinus rhythm is breaking through.

## Automaticity

Modern pacemakers are often equipped with some sort of automatic threshold measurement together with adjustment of amplitude/pulse width when needed. If the threshold value increases, the amplitude will automatically be increased to maintain safety margin. Different manufacturers have different solutions for this.

## Programming Amplitude and Pulse Width

When programming amplitude and pulse width, it is important to ensure that every delivered pulse leads to capture and to keep in mind that higher amplitudes or longer pulse widths will lead to higher current drain and ultimately decreased lifetime of the device. Also, the threshold value may

36

not be stable and may change over time. It is therefore necessary to program amplitude/pulse width with a certain safety margin to ensure that capture is still maintained if small changes in the threshold should occur. Two rules of thumb are commonly used when deciding safety margin. Both of these are based on the measured threshold:

2 x the amplitude threshold *or* 3 x the pulse width threshold

*Example:* The threshold is measured to 1 V@0.4 ms. The two rules of thumb give two possible combinations, either 2 V@0.4 ms or 1 V@1.2 ms. In clinical practice, pulse widths longer than 1 ms are most often avoided, and the same goes for amplitudes below 2 V. Therefore, in this example, 2 V@0.4 ms is the preferred choice.

The energy content of the pulse is determined by the combination of amplitude and pulse width. The safety margin reached by programming according to one of the rules above gives a certain margin in *percentage* for all possible thresholds, but the threshold itself doesn't really change in percentages. Rather, it is changing in volts or in parts of volts. A safety margin of twice the amplitude is accordingly much smaller for a threshold value of 0.5 V (programming of 1 V results in safety margin of 0.5 V) than for a threshold of 1.5 V (programming of 3 V gives a safety margin of 1.5 V). This is the reason why ventricular amplitudes are seldom programmed below 2 V (some clinics never go below 2.5 V), while the atrial amplitude may be programmed somewhat lower (1–1.5 V if the threshold permits). The fact that the atrial lead is more often not life-supporting makes a lower atrial safety margin more acceptable.

Within the first few weeks after the implantation of a new lead, a threshold rise may be seen. This is due to an inflammatory process triggered by the foreign body. This acute process commonly ceases within a month, and the first pacemaker follow-up is therefore planned six to eight weeks after implantation. The threshold value should be stable by then, and an optimization of the amplitude and pulse width can be safely performed. Before this first follow-up, these parameters are normally left at somewhat higher values (for example 3.5 V@0.4 ms) for newly implanted leads.

# Sensing

A pacemaker only stimulates when it is necessary to do so. To facilitate this behavior the pacemaker senses, via the implanted leads, the electrical signals of the heart chamber where the lead is placed. These signals are commonly called EGM signals (electrograms) and originate from the depolarization of the heart cells in close proximity to the electrodes of that lead. Once a signal is sensed, the pacemaker knows that a heartbeat has taken place and the next planned stimulation pulse is inhibited. For sensing to work properly, the sensitivity parameter needs to have the correct programmed value. This parameter is programmed in mV (millivolts), and it sets the lowest signal amplitude needed to be judged by the pacemaker as being a heart signal and inhibits the next stimulation pulse. It is easy to be confused by the terminology here, since a high sensitivity means a small value in mV (meaning that very small signals also will be detected), while a low sensitivity means a high value in mV. Hence, an atrial sensitivity of 0.3 mV is considered to be a high sensitivity, while 3 mV is considered to be low. When programming sensitivity, we optimize the value in order to sense all heart signals from the chamber where the lead is placed while at the same time avoiding sensing of extracardiac signals. Examples of extracardiac signals are muscle signals, external EMI and signals generated in the opposite heart chamber. If sensitivity is set too high, a phenomenon known as oversensing may occur. This could lead to inhibition of the stimulation pulse without a preceding intrinsic beat, and it may cause dizziness, presyncope or syncope. A sensitivity that is programmed too low may lead to an inability to correctly sense the intrinsic signals and thereby miss that stimulation is not needed. This is called undersensing and will lead to stimulation pulses into the intrinsic rhythm. That may seem harmless, but it could (although rarely) cause arrhythmias if the stimulation pulse hits the T wave (in the so-called vulnerable phase).

## Automaticity

It is quite common in modern pacemakers to have some sort of automatic adjustment of the sensitivity parameter. This automaticity is built on measurements of the sensed signals, which will be used to decide the sensitivity value. A proper safety margin can thus be obtained in spite of variations in the sensed signal amplitude.

## Programming Sensitivity

To be able to make a correct adjustment of the sensitivity value, a measurement of the EGM signal is mandatory. This measurement is performed automatically by the programmer and displayed in mV. Since EGM signals may vary a bit in amplitude, a certain safety margin is recommended when programming sensitivity. A safety margin of at least 2-3 times is commonly used. As an example, a P-wave amplitude of 1.5 mV may lead to a programmed sensitivity value of 0.5 mV (3x safety marginal). However, this rule of thumb may not be used single-handedly and must be used as one part in the decision process. In the atrium, the possible occurrence of atrial arrhythmias (mainly atrial fibrillation) needs to be taken into account. It is common to find that the EGM signals during atrial fibrillation are smaller in amplitude than those during sinus rhythm, and thus the signals require a higher sensitivity to be sensed correctly.

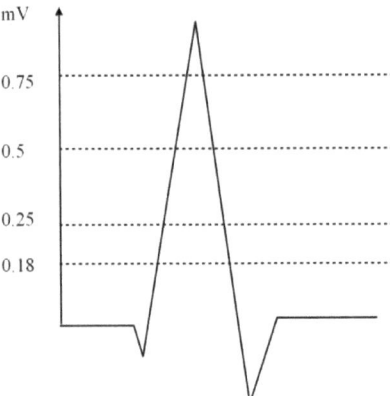

**FIGURE 4.10** The EGM signal with various sensitivity settings

When programming ventricular sensitivity, the signal is commonly strong enough to allow for a higher safety margin. If, for example, the R wave is measured to be 20 mV, a sensitivity value of around 4 mV may still be appropriate. To program a higher value could lead to undersensing (for example, of PVCs) but will not add to the safety against oversensing. Which value to program also depends on the programmed sensing polarity (see next section). Bipolar sensing polarity means less risk for oversensing, but the EGM amplitude is affected by the vector by which the signal hits the electrodes. A higher sensitivity is therefore desired in bipolar sensing polarity to avoid undersensing of PVCs. Unipolar sensing polarity leads to a higher risk of oversensing and a lower sensitivity is therefore needed.

# Polarity

To facilitate stimulation and sensing, two electrodes are required. During stimulation the electrical current is sent from one electrode to the other, and during sensing the difference in electrical potential is measured between the electrodes. The tip electrode of the lead is always used as one electrode, while the other electrode can be either the metallic pacemaker can (unipolar polarity) or a ring electrode placed proximally on the lead in the heart (bipolar polarity). Both polarities have their pros and cons, but bipolar leads are more often used today. If a bipolar lead has been implanted, the polarity may be programmed to unipolar or bipolar. With unipolar leads, there are no such possibilities since the ring from the bipolar lead is missing.

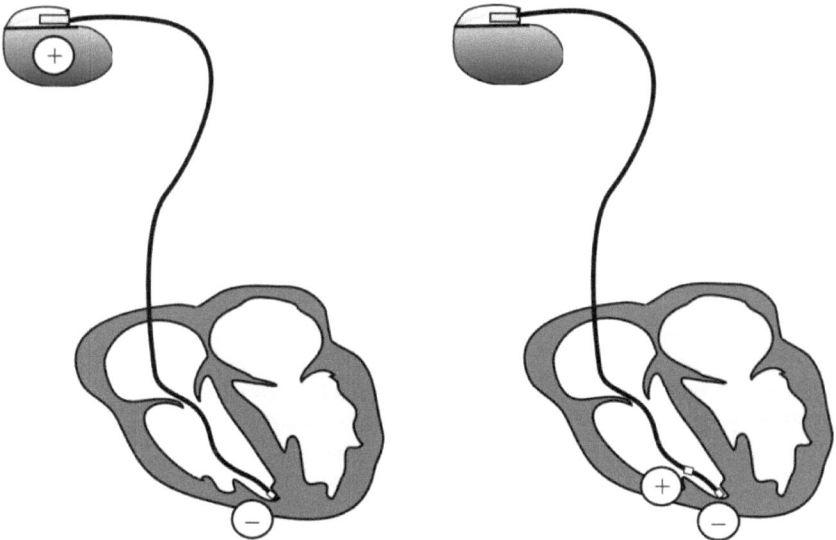

FIGURE 4.11 Unipolar polarity to the left and bipolar polarity to the right

# Pacing Polarity

The pacing polarity defines the way in which the stimulation pulse is delivered. For unipolar pacing, the metallic can of the pacemaker is electrically active and works as one electrode. Therefore, a disadvantage of unipolar pacing is the possibility to also stimulate the pectoral muscle (if that is where the device is placed), making the arm and shoulder twitch. An advantage of unipolar pacing is the comparatively long current path through the body, making unipolar pacing spikes clearly visible on surface ECG.

In bipolar polarity, pacing spikes may be more difficult to identify on surface ECG, but it has the advantage of not causing stimulation in the pocket. During implantation, or when exchanging an old device, bipolar pacing may be preferred since the system is stimulating the heart regardless of whether the pacemaker can is in the pocket or not. A unipolar pacing system stops stimulation when the pacemaker, being one of the electrical electrodes, is not in contact with the body. If a bipolar lead is damaged, it often starts working again when reprogrammed to unipolar polarity. However, this should not to be seen as a permanent solution, and after reprogramming it is important to closely follow that lead to ensure that the damage is not deteriorating to affect also the unipolar conductor.

*NOTE: When measuring sensing or pacing thresholds, it is mandatory to always do so with the device programmed to the polarity that will be permanently programmed when the patient leaves the clinic. Measured values can be markedly different depending on which polarity is used for the measurement.*

# Sensing Polarity

Sensing occurs when the difference in potential between the electrodes is higher than the programmed sensitivity in mV. The programmed sensing polarity influences the size of the sensed signal by the way the positive electrode (anode) is positioned. In unipolar sensing, the anode is positioned outside the heart (being the can) and signals that hit the lead tip will most likely not simultaneously hit the can. This gives the unipolar system a bit of an antenna effect, making it more sensitive to external noise (interference) which is more easily picked up. In bipolar sensing, the electrodes are positioned more closely together within the heart. The sensed heart signal corresponds to the difference in potential that results between the electrodes when the depolarization wave passes by. A depolarization wave that spreads over the heart tissue perpendicular to the electrodes, and thereby hits them simultaneously, will not result in a difference in electrical potential and will therefore not be sensed by the pacemaker (undersensing). It is important to take this into account when programming ventricular sensitivity, since PVCs spread by a different vector than measured R waves. The problem increases with decreasing tip–ring distances. However, the disadvantage must be balanced against the advantage of a decreased risk for interference. In the atrial channel, bipolar sensing polarity is nearly always used to avoid interference at the comparatively high atrial sensitivity. In the ventricle, the advantages of bipolar sensing are less prominent.

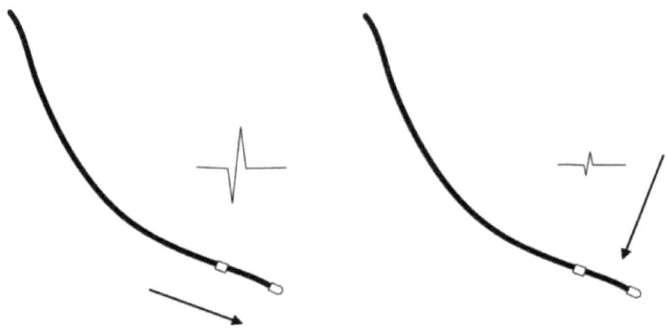

FIGURE 4.12 Vector-dependent sensing with bipolar polarity. Left: the heart signal is conducting along the lead body and hits the electrodes sequentially, leading to a large difference in potential and a high amplitude of the sensed signal. Right: The heart signal hits both electrodes simultaneously, leading to a small difference in potential and a low amplitude (if any) of the signal.

## Provocation Test

The use of unipolar sensing increases the risk of oversensing myopotentials since the anode, being the pacemaker can, is placed on the pectoral muscle. To ensure that myopotentials are not inhibiting stimulation, a muscle provocation test may be warranted. This is easily performed by asking the patient to press his/her hands together in front of the chest (like praying) to activate the pectoral muscle. At the same time, ECG and markers are monitored on the programmer screen and any sign of oversensing is noted. If oversensing is present, the sensing polarity should be changed to bipolar if possible or the sensitivity needs to be changed to a higher value (less sensitive). A decreased sensitivity must never lead to undersensing of the heart signals, however. Sometimes a suboptimal programming may still be necessary if reoperation to implant a bipolar lead is not desirable.

# Automaticity – Lead Monitor

Pacemaker leads are usually built with a coaxial design, meaning that the conductor/conductors are coiled around an empty core. Bipolar leads have an inner and an outer conductor coil with an inner insulation in between and an outer insulation on top. The inner conductor, which is used for unipolar pacing/sensing, is connected to the lead tip electrode. The outer conductor is connected to the ring electrode. This design ensures that the unipolar conductor of the lead is more protected and will most likely break at a later stage than the outer conductor if the lead is subject to damage. As a safety function for bipolar leads, modern devices can be programmed to constant monitoring of the lead impedance (electrical resistance) and, if signs of a lead failure are found, the device can be automatically switched from bipolar to unipolar (so-called lead monitor). Such a reprogramming will often ensure proper lead function for an extended time period and may even be life-saving for a patient with a partly damaged lead. This function should always be switched on when using a bipolar lead.

# Programming Polarity

For unipolar leads, bipolar polarity is not possible due to the missing ring electrode. Bipolar leads are usually programmed to bipolar sensing and pacing polarities. Historically, bipolar leads were often programmed to bipolar sensing and unipolar pacing, especially for the ventricular channel. This programming was based on the fact that early bipolar leads did not have the same reliability as unipolar leads. To ensure pacing in the ventricle, unipolar pacing polarity combined with the advantages of bipolar sensing was therefore popular. Today there are no significant differences in the performance of unipolar and bipolar leads, so this way of programming is less commonly seen.

Bipolar sensing is advantageous to avoid oversensing. Unipolar sensing is used when a disadvantageous vector of the sensed signal (usually PVCs) is causing undersensing. Unipolar pacing spikes are more easily noted on the ECG than bipolar ones. Unipolar polarity can also be used with bipolar leads when the outer conductor is failing.

# Single-Chamber Parameters

## Single-Chamber Lower Rate

A pacemaker could, in a simple way, be described as a computer, or even simpler, as a number of counters. While we think in terms of rate (beats/minute), the counters in the pacemaker count the number of milliseconds (ms, 1/1000 of a second) between each event (heartbeat). Programming a lower rate of 60 min$^{-1}$ (per minute) thereby corresponds to 1000 ms, which equals one second between every beat. The single-chamber pacemaker will never allow a longer time period than that to pass between heartbeats. To accomplish this, a lower rate counter starts counting every time the pacemaker senses a spontaneous heartbeat or delivers a stimulation pulse. The counter is reset and restarted on every sensed heartbeat. If the counter reaches its programmed value (corresponding to the programmed rate), a stimulation pulse is delivered and the counter restarts. This behavior continues throughout the lifetime of the device. During spontaneous rhythms faster than the programmed lower rate, the pacemaker will stay inhibited (the counter is reset at every beat without delivering a pulse). When the spontaneous rate falls below the programmed lower rate, the pacemaker will stimulate at that rate.

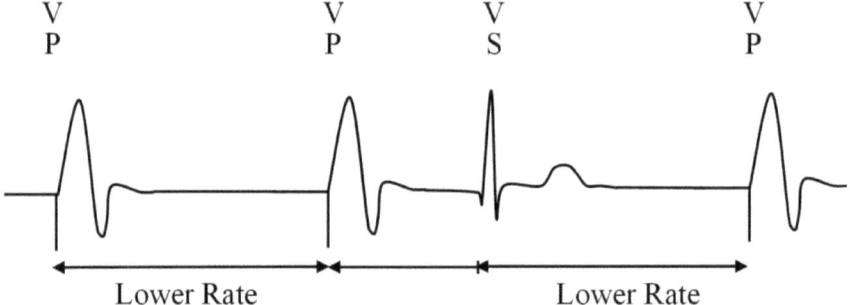

FIGURE 5.1 ECG with visualized lower rate timer

## Programming Single-Chamber Lower Rate

When programming lower rate, there are several factors to take into consideration. The most obvious one is perhaps also the most difficult to judge, namely which rate will be hemodynamically advantageous for this specific patient? The decision is most often not based on any measurement but on experience alone. The age of the patient must be taken into account (children have a higher heart rate than adults) as well as any comorbidity. Sometimes a lower rate of 70 $min^{-1}$ is recommended for patients with paroxysmal atrial fibrillation. Some evidence exists in literature that a stimulation rate of 70 $min^{-1}$ may suppress episodes of AF[1].

---

[1] Pacing Clin Electrophysiol. 2003 Sep;26(9):1841-8

The programmed pacing mode is also of importance. In VVI and AAI mode, an optimized lower rate is more important than in DDD or rate-responsive modes (sensor function). This is due to the fact that in VVI/AAI, no rate variation can be provided by the device, hence leaving the patient with the same heart rate in both rest and activity. It is also important to keep in mind that a programmed rate just above the intrinsic rate will lead to a larger percentage of pacing and consequently a shorter battery life. If the programmed rate is below the intrinsic rate for larger parts of the day, less pacing and a longer battery life can be achieved.

# Hysteresis

Hysteresis is programmable in most single-chamber pacemakers. A pacemaker with programmed hysteresis can be said to work with two separate sets of lower rates: one for pacing and one for sensing, where the pacing rate is higher than the sensing rate. Sensing is allowed below the lower rate, down to a programmable hysteresis rate. If the intrinsic rate falls below the hysteresis rate, the pacemaker will start stimulating at the lower rate. Hysteresis was more often used in early single-chamber devices to avoid symptoms from alternating stimulation and spontaneous rhythms.

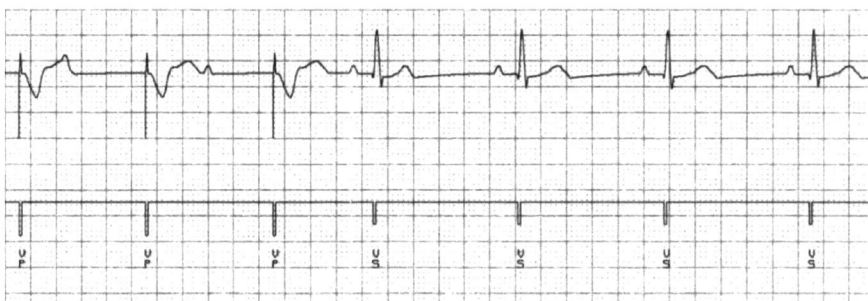

**FIGURE 5.2** ECG illustrating hysteresis function with a prolonged lower rate interval after a sensed event

## Programming Hysteresis

Hysteresis is programmed differently depending on the pacemaker manufacturer and model. However, the most common way is to program a certain hysteresis rate, usually 10 to 20 beats below the lower rate. In older models, hysteresis was sometimes programmed in milliseconds or even as a percentage of the lower rate interval.

# Night Rate

Modern pacemakers commonly allow for a lower stimulation rate at night. This could, for example, be achieved by programming the times between which a night rate should be active. At the programmed bedtime, the pacemaker slowly decreases the lower rate until the night rate is reached. The night rate will then be gradually increased at a pre-set time in the morning. Night rate is more often used in single-chamber devices and offers a way to provide a higher heart rate during the day and a lower one at night, which is physiologically advantageous. For patients with AV block, an intact sinus node and a DDD pacemaker, night rate is usually redundant. For this patient population, the sinus node will provide the rate and thereby a physiologic rate can be maintained with natural variations over day and night.

## Programming Night Rate

For many patients, night rate is not really important. Some patients however, do improve with a lower rate during the night, which can then be achieved by programming the night rate to *on*.

# Single-Chamber Refractory and Blanking Periods

For the pacemaker to work properly, it is important that each heartbeat is only sensed once. This is facilitated by turning the pacemaker input amplifier off for a short time after each sensed and paced event and is called the refractory period. The first part of the refractory period is called the blanking period, during which the amplifier is completely switched off and no sensing is possible. After the end of the blanking period, a sensed signal in the refractory period is not allowed to affect the lower rate timer. In this way the refractory period is in some ways similar to the refractory period of the heart cells and is also used as a safety feature to prevent fast, non-physiologic signals (noise) from inhibiting the pacemaker.

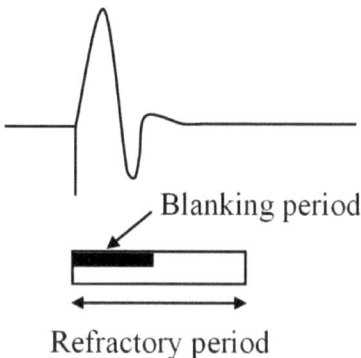

FIGURE 5.3 The refractory and blanking periods in the single chamber VVI device

If a signal is sensed during the refractory period, this will be restarted, meaning that repeated refractory senses may force the pacemaker to stimulate asynchronously at the lower rate until the noise ends, a function called noise reversion.

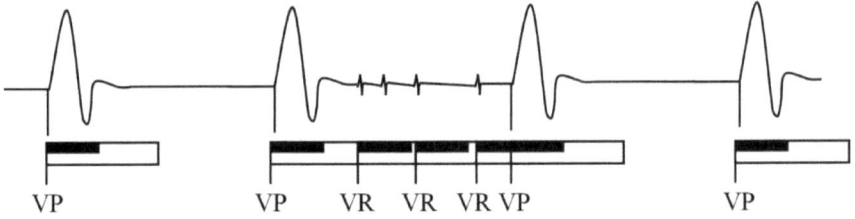

FIGURE 5.4 Noise Reversion during noise

# Polarization

When the pacemaker delivers a stimulation pulse, an electrical reaction around the electrodes is initiated. The lead tip, being the negative pole (cathode), will attract positive ions from the area around the tip. These positive ions will make it more difficult to push electrical current out through the tip, and the resistance that is built up increases with increasing pulse width. When the pulse is ended, the attracted ions will form a remaining electrical potential on the lead tip, called polarization. The polarization will decrease slowly or be reset by the pacemaker using a pulse with switched polarities, called a fast-recharge pulse. Some lead models build more polarization than others. A low-polarization lead may be necessary for some pacemaker features to work.

# Far-field Signals

When the pacemaker senses the heart activity in form of the EGM, it is desirable that the only signals sensed are those initiated in the chamber where the lead is placed. Unfortunately it is not uncommon for the atrial lead to, in addition to sensing atrial signals, also pick up the QRS complex from the ventricles. This signal, called far-field, consists of the summed ECG signal that is being registered between the atrial electrodes.

This signal can often be clearly differentiated from the P wave by its lower-frequency content and commonly also by its lower amplitude. A far-field QRS looks very much like a surface ECG, with broader complexes than the intracardiac ones and commonly also with a visible T wave.

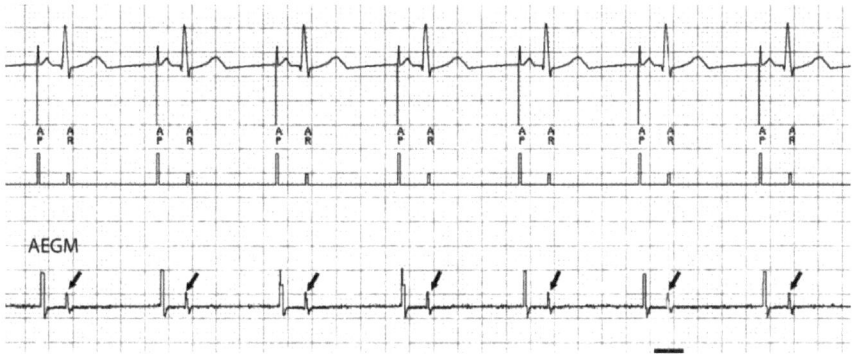

FIGURE 5.5 Far-field signals from the ventricle can clearly be noted on the atrial EGM

## Programming Single-Chamber Blanking and Refractory Periods

The blanking period, commonly 150–200 ms, is not often reprogrammed in VVI mode. It needs to cover the polarization signal and possible T waves. Each ventricular event must only be sensed once.

When programming blanking and refractory periods for the AAI pacemaker, one has to take into consideration possible far-field signals from the ventricle. Such signals should preferably be covered by the blanking period, but if sensed very late it may be enough if they are covered by the refractory period. This is important in order not to allow

53

those signals to reset the lower rate timer and by doing so allow for a heart rate below the lower rate.

# Dual-Chamber Parameters

## Dual-Chamber Lower Rate

In dual-chamber pacing, the lower rate is the rate limit at which the pacemaker is activated. When sinus rhythm is above the lower rate, atrial pacing is inhibited. Once the sinus rhythm falls below the lower rate, the pacemaker will start stimulating the atrium at the lower rate. During dual-chamber stimulation and sinus rhythm in the DDD mode, the heart rate varies in a physiologic way and a lower lower rate may be called for so there is no interference with the intrinsic rhythm. An increase in heart rate during exercise may be achieved either by following the sinus rhythm (DDD) or by rate-responsive pacing based on the sensor (DDDR).

### Programming Dual-Chamber Lower Rate

Recommendations are similar to those for single-chamber lower rate, with the exception for patients with adequate sinus rhythm. In these patients, a lower lower rate may be chosen.

# AV Delay

To allow for the best possible hemodynamic, correct programming of the AV delay is essential. With the different AV delay parameters available, we can control the PQ interval and directly influence the heart function. It is important to remember that the programmed AV delay never equals the resulting PQ interval, and that it is the PQ interval that is of importance. There are several factors influencing the difference between the programmed AV delay and the resulting PQ interval. The more important ones are described below, along with suggested programming strategies to compensate for these.

Since the beginning of the twenty-first century, several studies have been published showing that unnecessary stimulation of the ventricle may lead to an increased risk of developing atrial fibrillation as well as needing hospitalization due to heart failure[2]. It is therefore important to find an AV delay resulting in as little unnecessary ventricular pacing as possible. This is especially true for patients with already-existing heart failure. Unnecessary pacing in patients without AV block, or with intermittent blocks, can be prevented by prolonging the AV delay to promote intrinsic AV conduction whenever possible. However, it is not completely clear how programming of very long AV delays influences the risk of atrial fibrillation or heart failure. Too long PQ intervals are hemodynamically disadvantageous and should also be avoided.

## AV Delay for Sensed and Paced Atrium

To achieve the same PQ interval, whether the pacemaker is pacing or sensing the atrium, two different AV delays are programmable: one

---

[2] Circulation 2003;107;2932-2937

starting on the atrial sensed event and another starting on the atrial paced event. Two different factors influence the optimal difference between the two. When sensing the atrium, there is a slight delay from the start of the P wave (usually by the sinus node) on surface ECG to the moment when the signal reaches the atrial lead (usually placed in the right atrial appendage). This delay causes the PQ interval to be slightly longer than the programmed sensed AV delay (SAV).

When stimulating the atrium, the opposite is true. Some patients may exhibit a marked delay from the stimulation pulse to the visible P wave on surface ECG. This phenomenon is referred to as spike-to-P delay, and it is not fully understood.

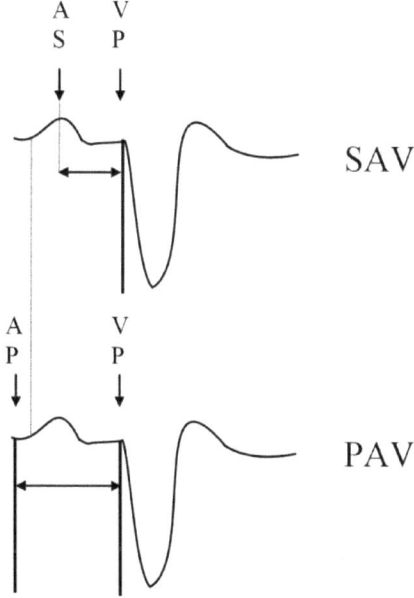

**FIGURE 6.1** Relation between SAV and PAV intervals

The spike-to-P delay is usually found to be only around 10 ms, but some patients present delays much longer than that. Spike-to-P delays up to 150 ms are certainly possible. For those patients, it is even more important to program a sufficiently long AV delay (PAV, Paced AV) to allow for an adequate PQ interval. As an example, a spike-to-P delay of 150 ms may lead to a programmed PAV of at least 300 ms to allow for a 150-ms PQ interval.

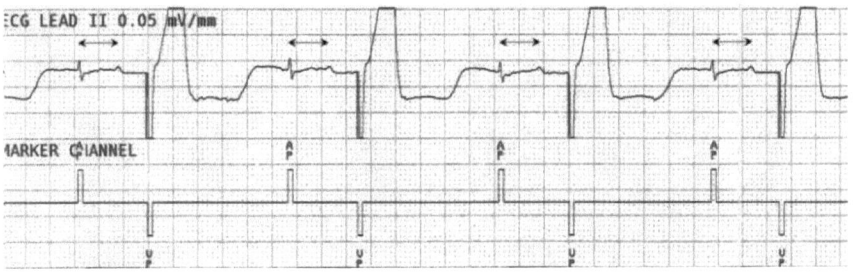

**FIGURE 6.2** ECG demonstrating a long spike-to-P delay of approximately 160 ms

If this phenomenon is not discovered and a short PAV is programmed, pacemaker syndrome may result when the atrium and the ventricle contract simultaneously. When this happens, the atria contract against closed valves due to the higher pressure in the ventricles. Blood from the atria will thus be pumped backward, out through the atrial inlet, which may result in dizziness and palpitations toward the neck. This may also, apart from the discomfort, lead to atrial fibrillation.

58

# Programming SAV and PAV

If no pronounced spike-to-P interval is noted, a common programming of SAV/PAV for AV block patients is 150/180 ms. Note that the PAV is always programmed longer than the SAV and that a normal offset between those is approximately 30 ms (with short spike-to-P intervals). If a delay from the atrial stimulation to the P wave on surface ECG is present, the PAV should be prolonged with at least that interval.

Since patients with sick sinus syndrome often are implanted with a dual-chamber system, it is important to ensure that spontaneous conduction is promoted if possible. A prolonged SAV/PAV, until no ventricular stimulation is delivered is preferred, although extremely long PQ intervals should be avoided for hemodynamic reasons. There are also automatic features available to promote intrinsic conduction (see below).

# Rate-Adaptive AV Delay

For patients with AV block, it is possible to mimic the way a healthy heart shortens the PQ interval during exercise. This is done by activating rate-adaptive AV, where the atrial rate is allowed to influence the length of the AV interval. Higher atrial rates will hence lead to shorter AV intervals. This will not only lead to better hemodynamics but will also allow the patient to reach higher heart rates during exercise (see also page 59: The pacemaker 2:1 block rate).

# Automaticity

Even before clinical trials had shown that unnecessary ventricular pacing was disadvantageous, many pacemaker manufacturers were developing algorithms to decrease ventricular pacing. In addition to the clinical advantages with spontaneous conduction (giving a more efficient heartbeat), less delivered stimulation prolongs battery longevity. Different manufacturers have different solutions, with the simpler versions being AV hysteresis with prolonged AV interval during ventricular sensing, while the more advanced algorithms automatically change the mode from AAI/R to DDD/R if needed (for example, Medtronic MVP and Sorin SafeR). If available, patients with intrinsic conduction should have such algorithms switched on.

# Ventricular Refractory Period

The ventricular refractory period in a dual-chamber pacemaker works much in the same way as it does in a single-chamber device. A timing window opens directly after ventricular sensing or pacing. Another sensed signal within this window is not allowed to affect the pacemaker's lower rate timer. Ventricular refractory period should cover the whole complex and, if present, also the T wave.

Also in the dual-chamber ventricular refractory period, a blanking period at the start of the refractory exists, where the input amplifier is switched off. However, this blanking period is most commonly not programmable.

## Programming Ventricular Refractory Period

Nominal setting is commonly around 230 ms. If no T-wave oversensing is noted, there is seldom any reason to change that setting.

# Atrial Refractory Period, PVARP

The atrial refractory period in the dual-chamber pacemaker is quite different from that in the single-chamber device. Firstly, the atrial chamber remains refractory during the AV interval, starting as an absolute refractory in the form of a non-programmable blanking period (during which the pacemaker input amplifier is shut off and possible heart signals will not be registered). This then continues as a relative refractory period with possibility for refractory senses. Secondly, what we usually refer to as the atrial refractory period starts on the following *ventricular* event (paced or sensed), i.e. at the end of the AV interval. The dual-chamber refractory period is therefore referred to as the post ventricular atrial refractory period, abbreviated PVARP. The PVARP also starts with a blanking period (post ventricular atrial blanking, PVAB) which is, as well as the PVARP itself, programmable. Sensed events in the PVARP will be marked as refractory senses and, as such, will not be allowed to start a new AV interval to initiate ventricular pacing.

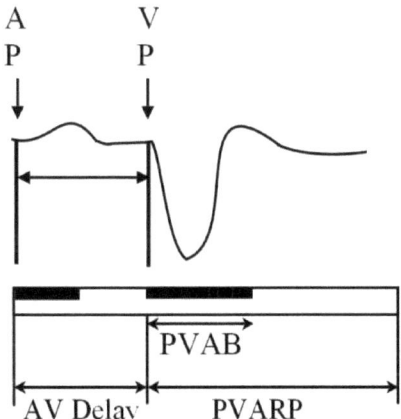

**FIGURE 6.3** The atrial refractory periods in DDD mode

The total atrial refractory period hence consists of the AV delay together with the PVARP. Together, these two limit the atrial rates that may be conducted to the ventricles by the pacemaker.

## Pacemaker 2:1 Block

When adding the programmed AV delay (SAV) and the programmed PVARP, the total atrial refractory period (TARP), in milliseconds, is achieved. This time period corresponds to the shortest interval between the P waves (highest rate) that may be conducted by the pacemaker from the atria to the ventricles. If faster atrial rates are present, every second P wave will fall into the PVARP and thus fail to start an AV delay. The ventricular stimulation rate will fall to half of that in the atrium, leading to a 2:1 block. If allowed to happen, 2:1 block is highly symptomatic and should always be avoided for rates that may be reached during exercise-induced sinus tachycardia.

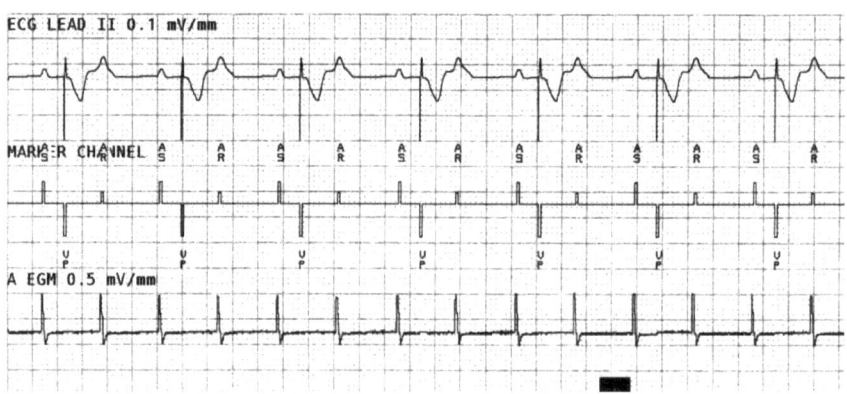

**FIGURE 6.4** The pacemaker reaches 2:1 block when the atrial rate has a P-to-P interval shorter than the TARP. Note the refractory sensed P waves (AR) on the marker channel.

The programmers often offer some help in the calculation of the pacemaker 2:1-block rate, but it can also be helpful to know how to do this calculation manually. One minute corresponds to 60 000 ms. When dividing 60 000 by TARP (in ms), the rate for 2:1 block is achieved.

Example: For a programmed AV delay of 150 ms and a PVARP of 350 ms, the TARP can be summarized as 150 plus 350 equals 500 ms.

$$60\ 000 \div 500 = 120\ \text{min}^{-1}$$

Since 120 min$^{-1}$ is quite a humble upper rate during exercise, we are forced to call in other functions to further shorten the TARP at higher rates to prevent the occurrence of 2:1 block. One of these functions, rate-adaptive AV, has already been described. Another useful function is to allow the pacemaker to also shorten the PVARP based on the atrial rate (auto PVARP).

It is important to remember that patients with intact AV conduction are not clinically affected by the pacemaker 2:1 block since every P wave, or atrial stimulation, will be conducted spontaneously by the heart. No rate drop will therefore be induced when the rate exceeds the TARP.

## Automaticity

Two different automatic functions can be used to avoid pacemaker 2:1 block at undesirably low rates. Both will, in different ways, affect the TARP, making it shorter when heart rate increases:

- Rate-adaptive AV (shortens the AV interval at higher rates)

- Auto PVARP (shortens the PVARP at higher rates)

# Programming PVARP/PVAB

Just like all the other programmable parameters, the PVARP/PVAB has been introduced to solve one or more possible problems. If the QRS on the atrial lead is large enough and has an EGM-like frequency content, it may be interpreted by the pacemaker as being an atrial signal (far-field sensing). If such a signal is sensed outside the refractory period, it will negatively affect pacemaker timing. It is therefore important that the PVARP (and preferably also the PVAB) covers the ventricular far-field signal. It is also important that the PVARP covers any retrograde P wave (VA conduction) to prevent pacemaker-mediated tachycardias.

## Retrograde Conduction and Pacemaker-Mediated Tachycardia (PMT)

Retrograde (VA) conduction is found in approximately two thirds of individuals with normal PQ interval[3]. The incidence is significantly lower in patients with antegrade (AV) conduction disturbances. For a pacemaker patient with a DDD pacemaker, retrograde conduction may lead to a problem commonly referred to as pacemaker-mediated tachycardia (PMT). This phenomenon is usually initiated by a PVC, when the cells in the AV node and in the atria are not refractory from a previous atrial event. The signal, originated in the ventricle, may then conduct backward over the AV node into the atria, starting an atrial contraction. If the signal is sensed outside the atrial refractory period, an AV interval will be initiated by the pacemaker and the ventricles will be

---

[3] Pacing Clin Electrophysiol. 1981 Sep;4(5): 548–562

stimulated at the end of this interval. The signal will again conduct backward and the loop created may be compared to a reentry tachycardia where the pacemaker acts as one half of the reentry circuitry and the retrograde conduction path as the other half. To prevent this from happening, the PVARP should be programmed longer than the retrograde conduction time. This may be tested by performing a retrograde conduction test where the pacemaker is programmed to VDI mode (VVI function with atrial sensing to aid measurements of possible retrograde conduction time). The programmed rate during the test should be higher than the intrinsic sinus rhythm to facilitate more room for conduction. ECG and EGM signals should be monitored carefully for a constant relationship between ventricular pacing and atrial sensing. If such a relationship is found, the interval between ventricular pace and atrial sense is measured, and the PVARP is programmed longer in order to cover the retrograde P waves. It should be noted that retrograde conduction may very well be intermittent and that the phenomenon cannot be ruled out even if it was not observable during the test.

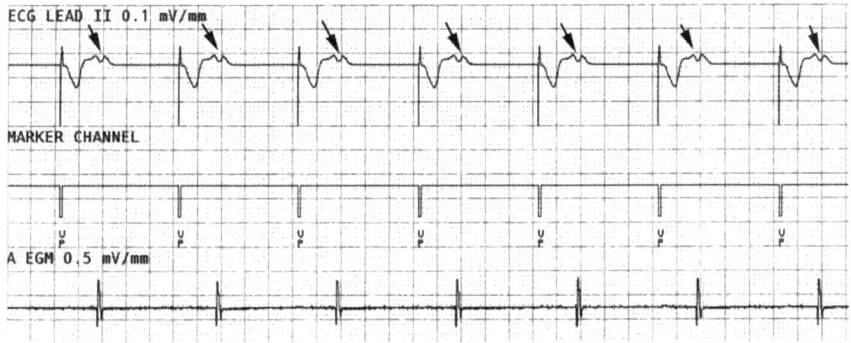

**FIGURE 6.6** Retrograde P waves emerging approximately 280 ms after ventricular stimulation

# Parameters Against PMT

PMT does not arise as long as the atrium and ventricle follow their normal sequence. In that way the atria and the AV node will be refractory during the propagation of the ventricular signal, which prevents retrograde conduction from occurring. To start retrograde conduction and PMT, the AV sequence hence needs to be broken. This is most commonly done by a PVC, but a few other mechanisms exist as well:

- Atrial exit block: The subsequent paced ventricular event may be conducted backward since the AV node and atrium are not refractory

- Atrial oversensing: Again, the subsequent paced ventricular event may be conducted backward since the AV node and atrium are not refractory

- Extremely long AV delays: Resulting in the end of atrial refractoriness before or during the propagation of the ventricular signal.

Two different algorithms are available to either prevent PMT from starting or to abort an already-ongoing PMT. Since the most common starter of a PMT is a PVC, most pacemakers automatically prolong the PVARP after a sensed PVC. This behavior ensures that any subsequent retrograde P wave falls within the PVARP and thus prevents PMT from starting. This feature may for example be called PVC response. To protect against other types of starters, another feature is commonly available to abort ongoing PMTs. This feature, PMT intervention, may be activated at a specific VA interval, or at a certain rate, and prolongs the PVARP as well.

## Programming Parameters Against PMT

If PVC response and PMT intervention are not programmed to the *on* position nominally, they should be switched on for most patients. The short pause in heart rhythm that may result from the prolonged PVARP, when a single P wave falls into refractory, very seldom causes any symptoms. In return, a good protection against PMT can be achieved without the need for a permanently long PVARP which would limit the maximum rate.

# Upper Tracking Rate

For most dual-chamber devices, it is possible to program two separate upper rates. One is the pacemaker upper tracking rate (UTR), defining the highest atrial rate that the pacemaker is allowed to track down to the ventricles. The other is the upper sensor rate, defining the highest sensor-driven rate that the patient can achieve (see page 80: Upper Sensor Rate). These two parameters are programmed separately and may have different values.

If the atrial rate reaches above the UTR, the ventricles are no longer allowed to follow every P wave, but they will maintain a rate close to the UTR. This behavior is made possible by means of a Wenckebach behavior with a varied degree of block. The pacemaker will keep track of the interval corresponding to the UTR and will not stimulate the ventricle until the UTR interval is reached. On ECG, a successive prolongation of the AV interval can be seen, with an occasional dropped beat before the sequence is repeated.

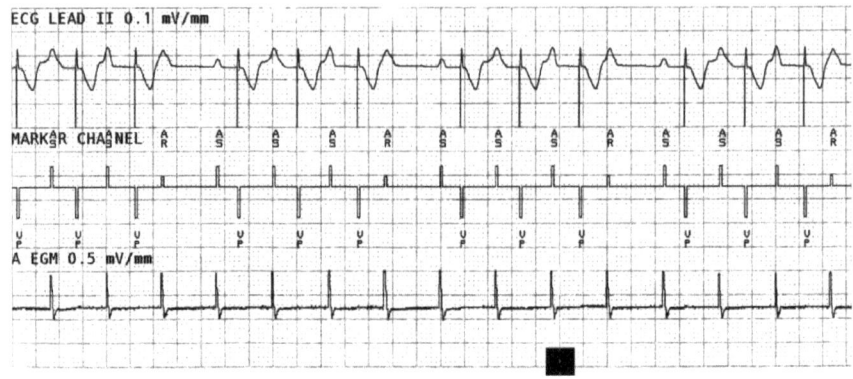

FIGURE 6.6 Wenckebach behavior when the intrinsic atrial rate reaches above the programmed UTR. Note the prolongation of the AV interval and the eventual dropped beat.

## Programming the UTR, AV Delay and PVARP

Since, in most cases, we don't know what rates the patient may achieve during strenuous exercise, and since blocking P waves during normal sinus rhythm are highly symptomatic, we need to take a few minutes with each patient to optimize programming of these parameters. A good start may be to make a simple calculation of the theoretical maximum rate for the patient. This is usually done as 220 minus the age of the patient. Many of our pacemaker patients have, in addition to advanced age, comorbidities or ailments limiting their exercise capacity. On top of that, many are taking beta blockers or other drugs in order to limit their heart rate. Once the maximum sinus rate has been estimated, the UTR is programmed to a rate slightly higher than that. With this completed, we then need to ensure that the 2:1-block rate is somewhat higher than the UTR.

68

# Ventricular Blanking and Ventricular Safety Pace

The phenomenon of far-field sensing of the QRS was explained in an earlier chapter. The opposite, far-field P waves, is not a problem as long as the ventricular lead is indeed placed in the ventricle. There is, however, another type of cross-chamber sensing that needs to be discussed, namely sensing of the atrial *stimulation pulse* on the ventricular channel. This is commonly referred to as crosstalk and may occur since the atrial stimulation pulse is in the range of 1.5 to 2.5 V and ventricular sensing occurs for signals in the millivolt region. A short blanking period is therefore launched in the ventricular channel each time the atrium is stimulated. This blanking period is extremely short (25-30 ms) and is only there to avoid crosstalk. If crosstalk nevertheless occurs (if ventricular blanking is too short), the consequences may be serious for pacemaker-dependent patients. The pacemaker will inhibit ventricular output, interpreting the signal as the ventricles already contracting, which may result in asystole. It is therefore important not to rely on blanking period alone but to also have other features to protect against crosstalk, which is described below.

One potential problem with a blanking period in the ventricle in close proximity to the atrial stimulation is the fact that the pacemaker will at that point start the AV interval, after which the ventricle will be paced. A PVC with an unfortunate timing could possibly hide in the blanking period, resulting in the following stimulation to hit in the T wave and the ventricular vulnerable phase. To minimize the risk for this behavior, the blanking period must not be programmed too long.

# Ventricular Safety Pace

Since a long ventricular blanking period may lead to undersensing of a PVC, and a too-short ventricular blanking period increases the risk of crosstalk, a separate security feature has been developed. This feature, ventricular safety pace (VSP), eliminates the risk for inhibition caused by crosstalk and, at the same time, takes into consideration that the sensed signal may originate from a PVC. When VSP is programmed on (and it should always be), the pacemaker will interpret any ventricular sense closely after an atrial pace as possible crosstalk. The next scheduled ventricular stimulation will therefore not be inhibited, but rather than stimulating the ventricle at the end of the AV interval, the pacemaker will shorten the AV interval to around 110 ms. If the sensed signal is not from crosstalk but an unfortunately timed PVC, stimulation will occur in the QRS and not in the vulnerable phase of the T wave.

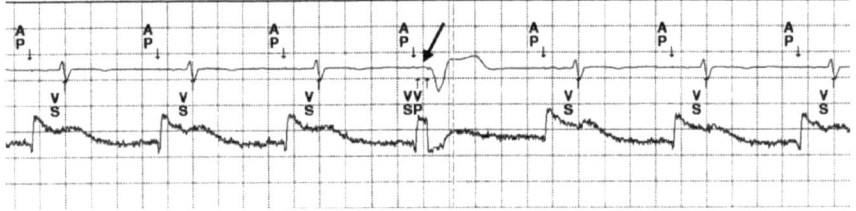

FIGURE 6.7 Ventricular safety pace initiated by crosstalk

# Programming Ventricular Blanking and Ventricular Safety Pace

Ventricular blanking is commonly programmed to 25 to 30 ms. There is no need to change that unless crosstalk is observed on ECG/markers. Ventricular safety pace should always be programmed on.

# Features for Atrial Tachycardia

Many patients treated with pacemakers also have atrial arrhythmias, either as a primary indication (i.e. slowly conducted atrial fibrillation), or as a secondary finding. Patients with sick sinus syndrome have a higher prevalence of atrial fibrillation than the general population, and since they commonly also belong to an age group with an increased AF risk (>75 years of age), it is important that the pacemaker can correctly detect, and adequately react to, atrial arrhythmias. The most commonly seen atrial arrhythmias are atrial fibrillation and atrial flutter, both quite easily detected by the pacemaker due to the high atrial rates. Atrial fibrillation can sometimes pose a problem for the sensing function, since signal amplitudes may be small and varying. This is important to take into account when programming atrial sensitivity. The value of the measured P wave is not giving any information about the amplitudes of the fibrillation waves, and hence standard sensitivity safety margin, set to the P wave, will not necessarily lead to correct sensing of the much smaller fibrillation waves. If the patient has a history of paroxysmal AF, but fibrillation waves cannot be measured during follow-up due to sinus rhythm, sensitivity should simply be programmed to a lower value (higher sensitivity) than would have been otherwised used.

Atrial flutter usually presents with much higher signal amplitudes, sometimes even higher than that of the measured P wave. The problem in atrial flutter is therefore not so much the amplitudes as the rate. Atrial flutter waves are often timed in such a way that every second signal falls within the PVAB (2:1-blocked flutter). In these cases, the pacemaker only detects every second signal and the mode-switch detection rate may not be reached. Instead of mode-switching, it tracks the arrhythmia at half its rate, which may be very symptomatic. Some devices have specific functions to look for this behavior, which will minimize the problem (for example, Medtronic Blanked Flutter Search).

# Mode-Switch

To prevent the pacemaker from tracking the high atrial rate during atrial tachycardia up to the MTR, it is important that the device be able to differentiate between non-physiologic tachycardia and fast sinus rhythm. This is accomplished by a function called mode-switch. When mode-switch is on, atrial rates exceeding a programmable detection rate will be detected as arrhythmia. The pacemaker will react to these arrhythmias by automatically changing the pacing mode from DDD/R (tracking) to DDIR (non-tracking). Once the rhythm converts back to sinus and the rate falls below the detection rate, the pacemaker will resume DDD/R mode. In this way the rhythm can also be kept low during atrial fibrillation and, by the use of a sensor (rate response), can even increase during exercise. This is immensely important since the hemodynamic capability may be largely impaired during atrial fibrillation.

## Programming Mode-Switch

Patients with paroxysmal atrial fibrillation/flutter should always have mode-switch on. In chronic AF, and with a DDD pacemaker, the mode may be reprogrammed to VVIR. In patients with no known atrial arrhythmias, the use of mode-switch can be discussed. Debuting arrhythmia may be less symptomatic with mode-switch on, and that in turn could prevent the patient from seeking medical attention. Eventual anti-coagulation treatment might thus be delayed, possibly resulting in embolic complications.

## Rate Regularization During Atrial Fibrillation

A non-negligible aspect of the symptoms experienced during atrial fibrillation originates from the irregular filling of the ventricles.

Pacemaker patients with an intact AV conduction may get some help from pacemaker functions regulating the rate, leading to a more consistent ventricular filling. These specific features (for example, Medtronic Conducted AF Response) continuously keep track of the average ventricular rate and stimulate at or around that rate. In this way the average rate is not increased but the rhythm, and thus the filling, becomes more regular. This, in turn, may reduce some of the symptoms.

## Prevention and ATP Therapies

At the end of the 1990s, there was strong belief that specific stimulation algorithms would have the power to decrease the number of AF attacks in patients with paroxysmal AF (so-called prevention algorithms). Many pacemaker manufacturers developed algorithms with the sole purpose of maximizing the amount of atrial pacing by continuously stimulating the atria just above the intrinsic rate. Later studies, however, have not been able to show any statistical difference in arrhythmia burden, and hence these algorithms are no longer commonly used. Even so, there is some clinical proof that a stimulation rate of $70 \text{ min}^{-1}$ could decrease the number of AF attacks, and it may very well be worth trying.

For a small number of patients with atrial reentry tachycardia in whom ablation has not been successful or is not possible, it may be suitable to try anti-tachycardia pacing (ATP) therapies. This is a pacing algorithm that may terminate arrhythmia by delivering fast overdrive pacing. At this point in time there are a very limited number of pacemaker models that offer ATP.

# Rate Response

For patients with chronotropic incompetence (inability to sufficiently increase heart rate), the implanted device needs to provide an increased heart rate during exercise. This feature, mimicking the function of the sinus node, is available in nearly all pacemakers on the market today and is visualized in the NBG code as an R (rate response) in position IV. Clinically, AAIR, VVIR, DDDR and DDIR (used during mode-switch) are commonly used.

Although the first pacemaker was implanted in 1958, it wasn't until 1985 that a pacemaker with a built-in sensor to adapt heart rate when needed became available on the market (Medtronic Activitrax). The sensor was a small piezoelectric crystal that recognized patient activity and converted mechanical energy to electrical signals from inside the can. The strength and frequency of the signals were proportional to the level of patient activity, and an algorithm was developed to convert increased sensor signal to increased heart rate. Similar sensors are still used today and have been shown to work reliably.

## Different Sensors

The goal for the rate response function is to mimic the function of a healthy sinus node as closely as possible. An ideal sensor would react on physical activity as well as psychological stress, fever, etc. Many different sensor types have been tested over the past years, but only a few are still in use. For a sensor to be suitable for use in an implanted pacemaker, it needs to have low energy consumption and it shouldn't need the implantation of a special lead (i.e. should be placed inside the pacemaker can). It should also give a balanced response to physical activity, be technically reliable, and be easy to understand and program. If it is also physiological (reacts to physiological stress), it is advantageous as well. Some of the physiological sensors that have been tested are minute ventilation (breathing), QT, oxygen saturation, and temperature. In spite of the advantages that a physiologic sensor may offer, they have all had to give way to the much simpler activity sensor which is dominating the market today. Combinations with dual sensors have also been tested, but these have not been found to offer much clinical advantage over the single sensor. For selected patients, however, dual sensors can be advantageous, and the most common combination today is that of activity + minute ventilation.


## The Activity Sensor

The most commonly used sensors on the market today are the activity sensors, most of which are built on a piezoelectric crystal. In modern pacemakers, this sensor is most often used as an accelerometer, detecting anterior-posterior motion. When the patient is at rest, the sensor does not generate any sensor signal and the pacemaker will stimulate at the programmed lower rate. During exercise/movement, the sensor will generate signals in proportion to the acceleration caused by the movement. The signals will be processed by the pacemaker microprocessor and converted into a rate increase proportional to the exertion. Since this type of sensor will give an immediate response to exercise, algorithms are needed to ensure that the rate acceleration/deceleration is performed in a physiologic manner. For example, if a patient jogs for an hour and then sits down directly after he stops exercising, the rate should not instantly return to lower rate even though the sensor signal drops to zero. A deceleration algorithm will ensure that the drop in rate is gradual, slowly bringing the rate down to the lower rate. There is also a need for an algorithm that, at the start of activity, gradually increases the heart rate to avoid an immediate raise to upper sensor rate if the patient is running for a few seconds to catch a bus. The algorithms responsible for rate acceleration and deceleration (when there is a difference between actual heart rate and sensor-indicated rate) are programmable and are commonly called acceleration and deceleration times.

## Activity Threshold

To assure that the heart rate is not influenced by eventual sensor signals at rest, programmability of a zero level is necessary. This is done by changing the activity threshold parameter which defines the zero level for the sensor, meaning the minimum level of sensor signal that is needed to start a rate increase. It is important to understand that the higher the activity threshold, the more sensor signal is needed to get a rate increase. The sensor is hence less sensitive with higher activity thresholds.

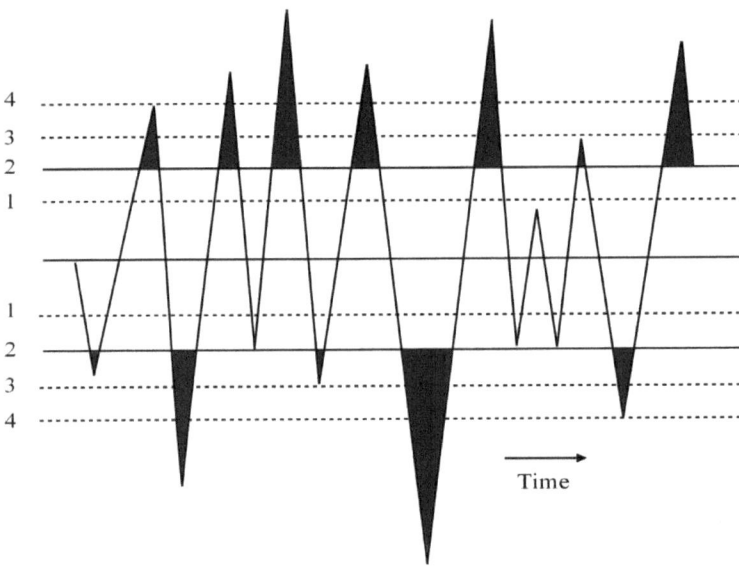

FIGURE 6.8 Activity sensor signal with thresholds 1-4 where 2 is the programmed threshold. Only signals higher than the programmed threshold are allowed to influence the sensor rate.

## Activity Slope

The activity slope defines the relation between the sensor signal and the rate increase. A higher sensor signal leads to a higher heart rate, and the slope defines what heart rate corresponds to a certain sensor signal.

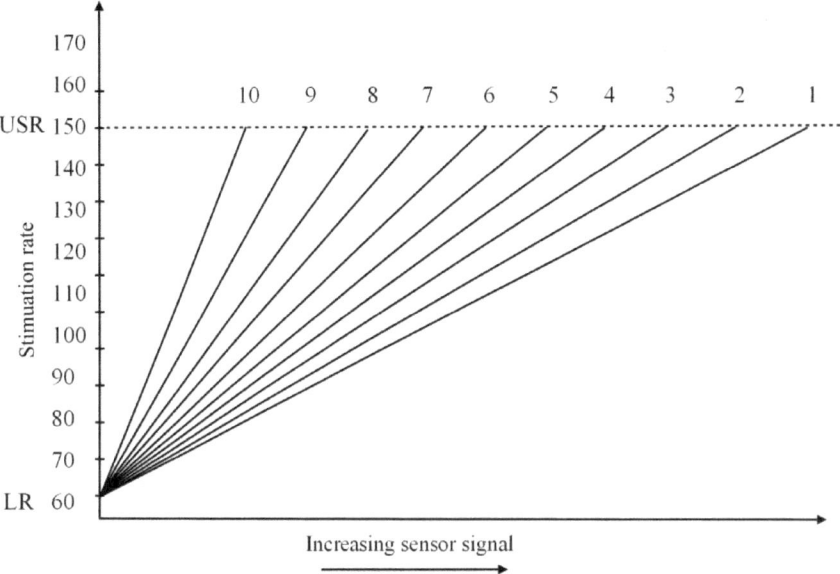

**FIGURE 6.9** Depending on the programmed slope, the patient will get a certain rate increase for a given sensor signal (workload)

As can be seen in the figure above, a steeper curve (higher number) will result in more rate increase than a less-steep curve for the same activity/sensor signal. If a higher heart rate for a given workload is desired, the curve is reprogrammed to a higher value.

Some pacemaker manufacturers have taken the algorithms one step further and incorporated dual slopes, where one slope defines the rate from lower rate to ADL (activities of daily living) rate and the other slope defines the rate from ADL to the upper sensor rate. This allows for fine-tuning of the rate response in a more physiologic way over a wider span of activities.

## Acceleration and Deceleration Times

As described earlier, the activity sensor will give an immediate response to a change in activity level. Since the physiological rate increase is gradual and not immediate, special algorithms are used to limit the speed at which the rate is allowed to change (decrease or increase). How fast the rate can increase is decided by the acceleration time (or reaction time) parameter, and the decrease time is decided by the deceleration time (or recovery time) parameter. While acceleration time is usually programmed in seconds, deceleration time is more commonly programmed in minutes. Some pacemakers even offer the option to adjust the length of the deceleration time automatically, depending on the length and strength of the exertion. A short rush to catch a bus will give a shorter recovery time than ten miles of running.

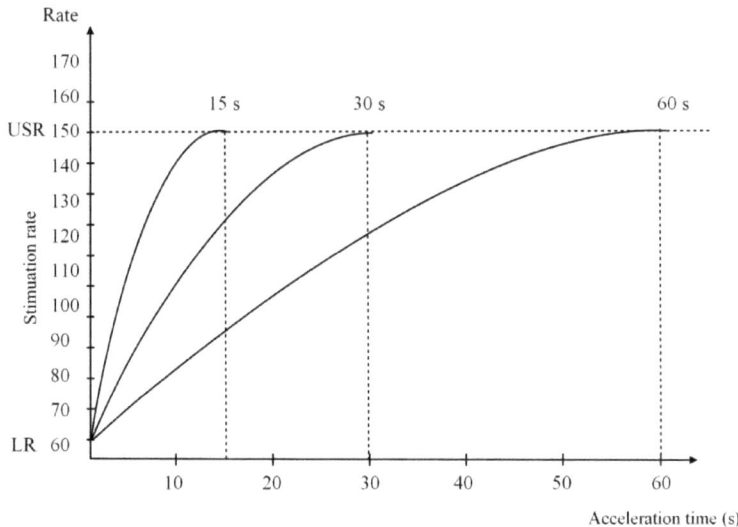

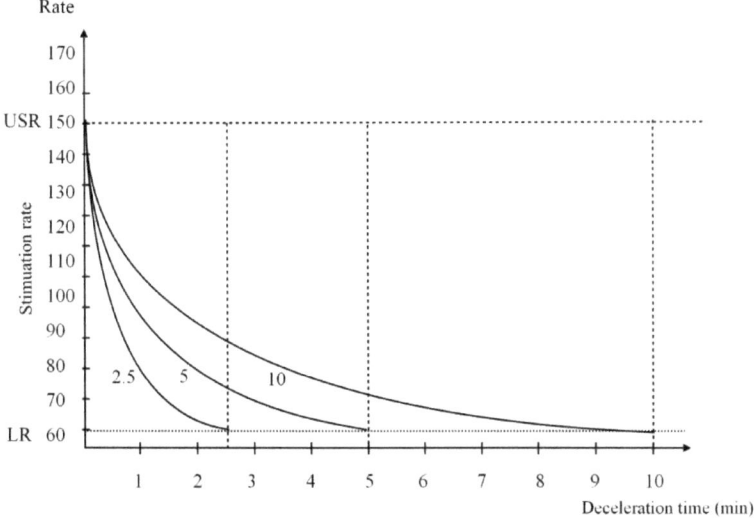

FIGURE 6.10 Acceleration (top) and deceleration (bottom) times

# Upper Sensor Rate

The heart rate, when driven by the sensor, is limited by the programmed lower rate and the programmed upper sensor rate (USR). Regardless of how strong the sensor signal may get, the pacemaker will never stimulate with a sensor-driven rate above the USR. However, it should be noted that the maximum tracking rate (MTR) may allow for intrinsic atrial rates to be tracked above the USR, if MTR is programmed to a higher rate than the USR.

# Automaticity

In the early rate-responsive devices, manual programming of slope and activity threshold was always necessary. In present devices, this is commonly done automatically by the pacemaker, which then evaluates the patient's activity level over several days and uses that information for sensor fine-tuning. Another advantage to this is that the sensor setting will adjust to changes in the patient's exercise levels and hence will simulate the healthy heart (for example, in fitness training).

# Evaluating Rate Response

Many pacemakers also offer the option to evaluate rate adaption during exercise through some form of programmer-driven exercise test. The patient is asked to perform a certain exercise for a specified number of minutes, such as walking in the corridor or climbing stairs. The heart rate during the activity is stored by the device and can be displayed afterward in, for example, a rate trend. In this way it is possible to make a judgment whether the resulting rate increase is optimal or if it needs to be adapted further. It is always a good idea to walk with the patient during the exercise to get a good idea of how strenuous the activity was. The graph will then give an idea how a specific reprogramming would influence the heart rate, and an optimal setting can be chosen.

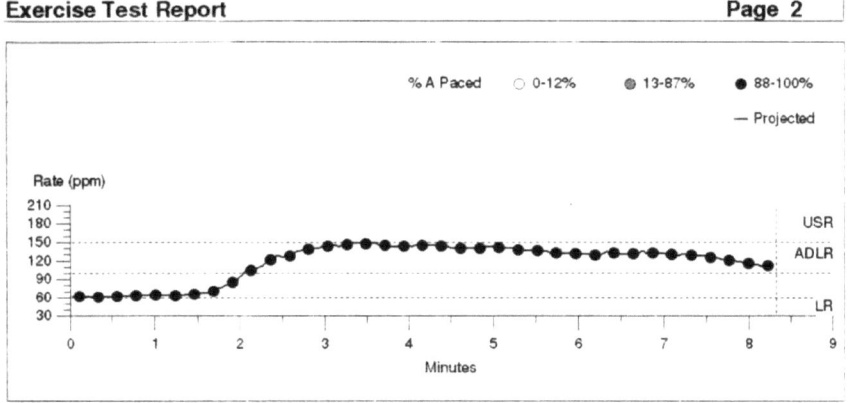

**FIGURE 6.11** Example of a graph from an exercise test with a Medtronic EnPulse device

# Programming Rate Response

One way to determine whether rate response needs to be programmed on or not is by looking at the rate histogram. This information, together with information about the patient's activity level, will give a rough idea of how the rate adaption is working. Naturally, one cannot expect rate variation to a larger extent for a very sedentary patient (for example, a patient in a wheelchair). If the rate distribution is scarce but the patient does not feel limited in daily life, there is usually no need for changes. Inversely, a normal rate histogram is not a guarantee of optimal rate-response programming. It is always important to take into account the patient's perceived exercise tolerance.

Programming of rate response varies for different systems, types of sensors, and manufacturers. The programming of the activity sensor,

81

however, is quite similar when it comes to activity threshold and slope. Automaticity may be very different between manufacturers, and individual assessment may be warranted to decide if it should be programmed on or if manual programming is a better choice.

# Follow-up Tools

There are several tools available to simplify interpretation of pacemaker function and facilitate troubleshooting of the system. To ensure that follow-up is performed safely and that pacemaker ECG interpretation is correct, use of a pacemaker programmer is necessary. Programmers vary from company to company, and in addition to showing the programmed parameters, they present data collected by the pacemaker as well as give access to ECG, EGM (electrogram) signals, and markers in real time. These tools are critical when interpreting the advanced pacemaker functions hosted by modern devices.

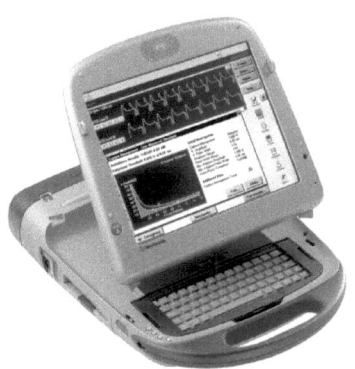

FIGURE 7.1 Pacemaker programmer model 2090 from Medtronic

83

# EGM

The EGM is the signal that the pacemaker receives from the heart via the lead. This signal directs the pacemaker function, and when the amplitude of the EGM signal is high enough, it will lead to sensing of that signal and inhibition of the next stimulation pulse. The EGM signal may also give additional information about the lead position in the heart, lead integrity and lead stability. It should prove very useful to become acquainted with the different EGM characteristics, especially during implantation.

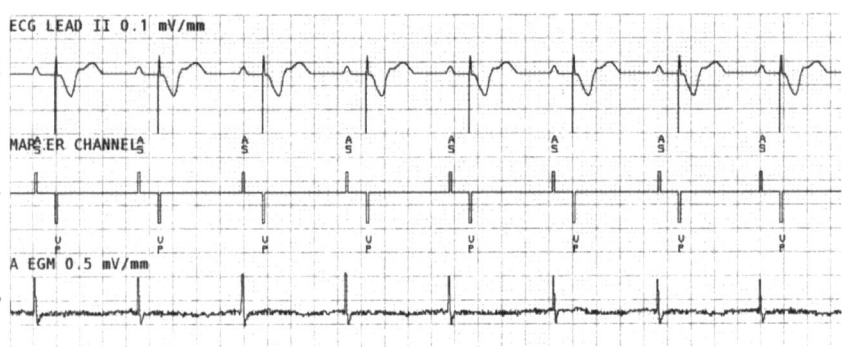

**FIGURE 7.2** The EGM signal (bottom tracing) may give additional information such as lead position and integrity

An EGM signal that is sensed from an electrode in contact with the heart wall is usually narrow and pointed. As opposed to the ECG, the EGM signal is not composed of as many summarized cells, but rather is the result mainly from a smaller amount of cells in close proximity to the electrode. The EGM signal is created when the polarization of the cells in the heart chamber where the lead is placed passes one of the electrodes. Depending on where the lead is placed in the heart, the EGM signal may

84

arise early or late on the surface ECG. For example, for a lead placed in the right ventricular apex, the ventricular signal is sensed quite late compared to the start of the QRS on surface ECG.

The morphology of the EGM signal also gives important information about lead position. A dislodged lead, or one that is perforated, gives a different signal morphology than a lead placed against the heart wall. In those circumstances, ECG-like signals with widened complexes and clearly visible T waves may be seen. This would be important to notice during troubleshooting as well as during implantation.

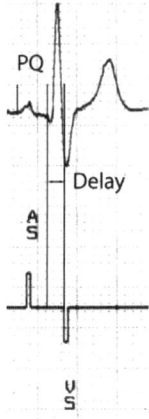

FIGURE 7.3 Late sense due to lead placement in the right ventricular apex. Approximate PQ time 160 ms, and time between AS and VS approx. 200 ms. The delay from start of QRS to VS is in this example approx. 40 ms.

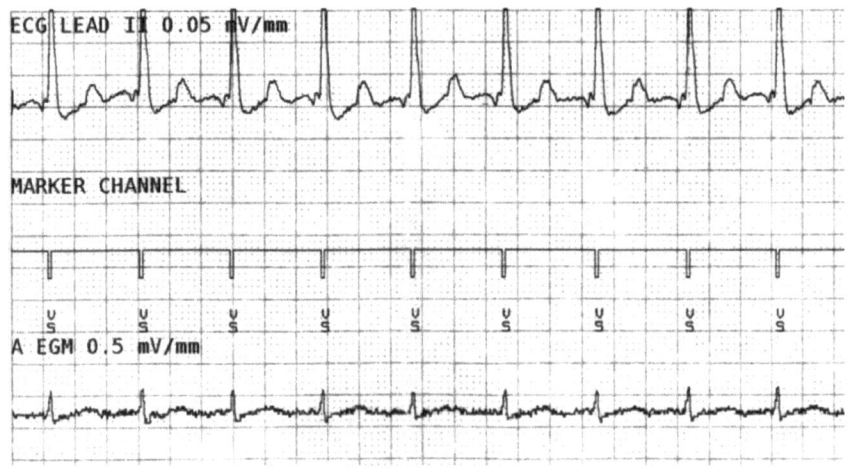

**FIGURE 7.4** Dislodged atrial lead free-floating in the ventricle in a dual-chamber device. Note the ECG-like morphology of the atrial EGM that coincides with QRS on surface ECG. The fact that no sensing occurs on the atrial lead on the ventricular signals is due to the PVAB started in the atrium at each ventricular event.

By looking at the atrial EGM signal, one also gets an indication whether far-field signals from the ventricle may be problematic. It is also important to note any large variations in signal amplitude and to compare the amplitude of conducted R waves with the amplitude for eventual PVCs. The information is used when choosing sensitivity as well as sensing polarity.

# Marker Channel

As described earlier, modern pacemakers are extremely advanced with thousands of programming possibilities, including many automatic features. To allow us to safely interpret the pacemaker ECG that results from treatment, we need the pacemaker to communicate what it is doing at any given moment. This is done via the marker channel. Together with the ECG and EGM, the pacemaker shows symbols for pacing and sensing as well as timing intervals in milliseconds. The symbols used differ somewhat between manufacturers. Most commonly used are the symbols AS (atrial sense), VS (ventricular sense), AP (atrial pace), VP (ventricular pace), AR (atrial refractory sense), and VR (ventricular refractory sense). These symbols are used by Medtronic, Boston and newer St. Jude Medical devices. The markers P (P wave), R (R wave), A (atrial pace) and V (ventricular pace) also exist on older St. Jude Medical devices.

# Diagnostic Features

Pacemakers of today often include a variety of diagnostic functions. Data is continuously gathered and stored to provide as much information as possible about how the system has been working since the last follow-up. This data is displayed on the programmer during the follow-up. Collected data may be divided into clinical data (such as arrhythmias, conduction times and HF data) and system data (such as threshold values, sensing amplitudes, lead impedances and battery data). Data may be displayed as histograms, trends or numerical values. EGM signals may also be stored (for example, during arrhythmias) to facilitate diagnosis.

When looking through stored data, it is important to remember that not all devices present data in the same way. It is recommended that practitioners take the time to understand stored data for the systems used in their clinic. With some experience, it becomes possible to recognize certain patterns in the diagnostics as being signs of specific problems.

Most data will be reset automatically after follow-up, with the exception of some long-term trends. However, some manufacturers demand that reset be performed manually.

# Event Counters

Event counters are used to show the percentage of sensing and pacing. This is commonly done using the marker symbols.

**Since Last Session**
25-Aug-2010 to 05-Oct-2010
41 days

| | |
|---|---|
| **Total VP** | 99.7 % |
| **AS-VS** | 0.3 % |
| **AS-VP** | 83.0 % |
| **AP-VS** | < 0.1% |
| **AP-VP** | 16.8 % |

> 5% of AS may be due to FFRW

FIGURE 8.1 Event counters showing how the pacemaker has been working since the last follow-up session

Counters may also be used in arrhythmia diagnostics, such as number of episodes, length of episodes, start times, etc., or to show the number of PVCs or PACs since the last session.

# Heart Rate Histograms

The most elementary form of diagnostics, and the form that has been available the longest, is the heart rate histogram. This histogram displays the rate distribution separately for each heart chamber, commonly divided into paced and sensed events at the different rates. The rate histogram gives information about the patient's chronotropic competence (or incompetence). Every patient has his or her own individual rate distribution, influenced by age, activity level, possible comorbidity and medications.

**Atrial Long Term Histogram**

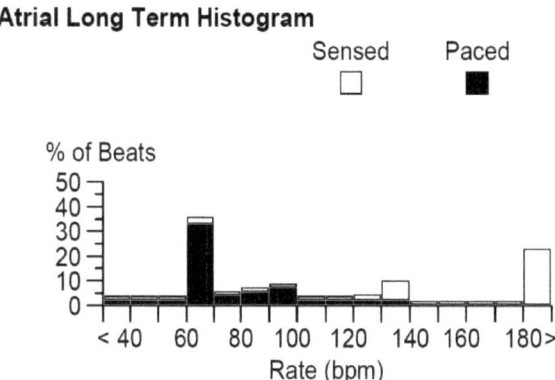

FIGURE 8.2 Rate histogram from a Medtronic Adapta, showing atrial rate distribution since the last follow-up. Note the bin to the right (>180 min⁻¹) illustrating atrial fibrillation in this patient.

In the atrial rate histogram, arrhythmias may be found as a registration of rate bins in the higher rates. However, it is important not to be fooled by sensing of far-field signals that may have the same appearance.

Histograms are built up exclusively by intervals from that one channel, which sometimes causes some confusion. If, for example, very low rates are seen in the atrial histogram, this is normally caused by the lower rate timer being reset on a PVC, with a compensatory pause in the atrium as the result.

# Sensing and Threshold Trends

For the pacemaker to work correctly, it is important that the sensing and pacing parameters be programmed to optimal values. In older models, measurement and programming of these parameters could only be done at the in-clinic follow-up session. As described earlier, modern pacemakers can often make these measurements and adjustments automatically while the patient is ambulatory. The results from the tests can in some models be displayed as long-term trends. These are very useful, both in evaluating pacemaker function at the in-clinic follow-up and during troubleshooting of possible lead problems.

# Atrial Sensing Trend

Variations in amplitude of the atrial signals are usually due to atrial fibrillation (with varying or small fibrillation waves). Variations could also be seen due to sensing of far-field signals from the ventricle, which will have different amplitudes than that of the P waves. Since bipolar sensing is used almost exclusively in the atrium, some variations in amplitudes may be caused by varying vectors in the signal propagation.

# Ventricular Sensing Trend

Amplitude variations in the ventricular channel are mostly seen due to the bipolar sensing configuration (PVCs with a different vector), and variation tends to be smaller in unipolar sensing. If T-wave oversensing is present, this will be registered as amplitude variations as well.

**P-Wave Amplitude    03/15/10 2:05 PM - 10/05/10 2:05 PM**

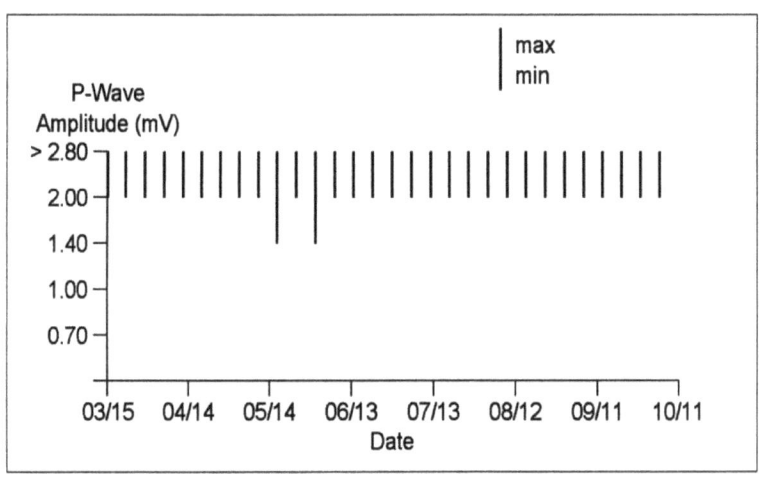

FIGURE 8.3 Example of an atrial sensing trend from a Medtronic Adapta

# Ventricular Threshold Trend

Many modern pacemakers have some sort of automatic ventricular threshold measurement. For these systems, there is usually also some kind of trending available, to show threshold variations over time. Even though these measurements tend to be both accurate and safe, there is always a small risk that the measurement results in a threshold value that is too high. Varying and/or high threshold values from the automatic features should always lead to thorough manual measurements to exclude that it is the measuring method, rather than the threshold itself, that is the problem.

91

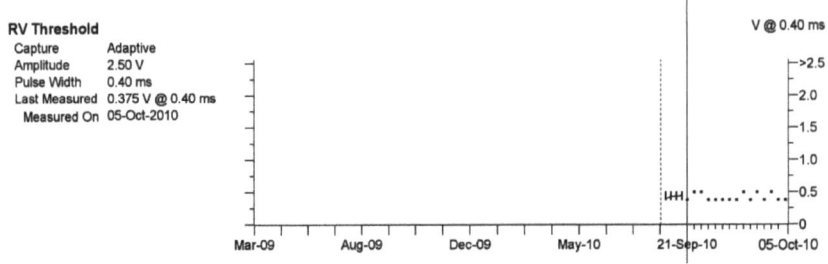

**FIGURE 8.4** Ventricular threshold trend from a Medtronic EnSura DR MRI

## Atrial Threshold Trend

Some companies offer pacemakers with automatic threshold measurements also in the atrium. These measurements are done in different ways by different companies, and it is therefore difficult to give any general advice on how to judge these data. Naturally, no measurements can be taken during atrial fibrillation/flutter.

## Arrhythmia Diagnostics

Patients with sick sinus syndrome are known to have a higher prevalence of atrial fibrillation than the general population. Patients in the age group most commonly treated with pacemakers (>70 years of age) have a higher risk of developing atrial fibrillation than younger individuals. Functions that adequately detect and react to arrhythmias have been discussed earlier in this book, and those functions can commonly also provide diagnostic features to evaluate arrhythmia burden, type of arrhythmia, treatment outcome, etc. Thus the pacemaker can provide important information that would otherwise be difficult to obtain without long-term ECG registration. Information is readily available regarding the

92

frequency of AF episodes (also those that are not symptomatic), the length of those episodes (which can help in deciding whether to use anti-coagulation or not), as well as ventricular rate during AF (to find out if rate regulation is needed). It is also possible to look at stored EGM signals from the time of the arrhythmia to determine start mechanisms and to separate clinical arrhythmias from oversensing or lead issues. It is common that the larger part of the pacemaker memory is used for this purpose. Even though atrial arrhythmias are more commonly seen, it is also important for the device to store episodes of ventricular arrhythmias for consideration.

|  | Prior Session<br>14-Dec-2009 to<br>25-Jan-2010<br>42 days | | Last Session<br>25-Jan-2010 to<br>11-Oct-2010<br>9 months | |
| --- | --- | --- | --- | --- |
| **AT/AF Summary** | | | | |
| % of Time AT/AF | 0.0 | % | 0.3 | % ↑ |
| Average AT/AF time/day | 0.0 | hours/day | <0.1 | hours/day ↑ |
| Monitored AT/AF Episodes | 0.0 | per day | 0.1 | per day ↑ |
| Treated AT/AF Episodes | 0.0 | per day | 0.0 | per day |
| Pace-Terminated Episodes | 0.0 | % | 0.0 | % |
| % of Time Atrial Pacing | 67.6 | % | 62.8 | % ↓ |
| % of Time Atrial Intervention | 0.0 | % | 0.0 | % |
| AT-NS (>6 beats) | 0.0 | per day | 0.3 | per day ↑ |

**Since Last Session** 25-Jan-2010 to 11-Oct-2010

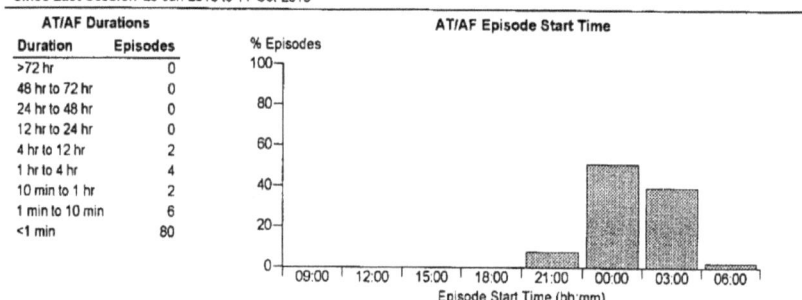

| AT/AF Durations | |
| --- | --- |
| Duration | Episodes |
| >72 hr | 0 |
| 48 hr to 72 hr | 0 |
| 24 hr to 48 hr | 0 |
| 12 hr to 24 hr | 0 |
| 4 hr to 12 hr | 2 |
| 1 hr to 4 hr | 4 |
| 10 min to 1 hr | 2 |
| 1 min to 10 min | 6 |
| <1 min | 80 |

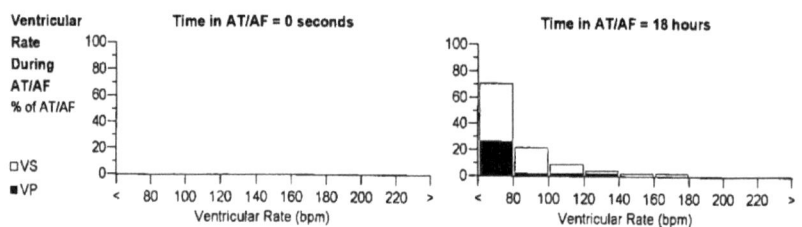

FIGURE 8.5 Example of arrhythmia diagnostics from a Medtronic EnRhythm

94

# Measured Values

Apart from measurements and data stored to facilitate clinical assessments, the system also presents information concerning its technical integrity as well as its battery status. These kinds of data used to be available only at follow-up but can now be measured automatically, sometimes several times per day, and be presented as trends. The most important of those trends is, according to the author, the lead impedance trend. Since the lead is always the weakest link in the system (a pacemaker very rarely stops working, except for at full battery discharge), it is important to continuously monitor the lead. Different systems have different solutions for this.

# Lead Impedance and Trends

The resistance in the electrical circuit during stimulation of the heart is called lead impedance. Hence, it is not the impedance in the lead itself as one might think, but the impedance in the total circuit (including the connection between pacemaker and lead, conductor impedance, etc.). The impedance, measured in Ohms, is normally found in the range of 400 to 1000 Ohms. The impedance value is affected by several factors, with the lead design being the most important one. Another factor affecting impedance is lead placement. Different placements in the same patient with the same lead may lead to different impedances. Different patients will have different impedances, and variations may be seen with relation to certain medications, electrolyte imbalance, etc. Average lead impedance in the atrium is also lower than that in the ventricle when using the same lead model. An ideal lead should have a high impedance together with a low stimulation threshold and good sensing. This is achieved by designing the lead in such a way that the larger part of the impedance is found in the interface between the stimulation electrode and the heart. In this way the amount of wasted power is low since most of the energy is used where it is needed (to stimulated the heart) and not for other reasons (for example, to heat up the conductor).

Pacemaker current consumption, and thereby battery longevity, is highly dependent on lead impedance. The higher the impedance, the lower the current for a given amplitude. The current consumed in each pulse can be calculated by using the law of Ohm:

$$Voltage = Impedance * Current$$

A lead with high impedance is therefore preferred over one with a lower value.

The most common problems seen in pacemaker treatment are related to the lead. Lead dislodgment during the first weeks after implant is not uncommon, and leads that have been implanted for a while may develop insulation damage or conductor break. Since it is not possible to design a lead that will function eternally in the hostile environment of the body, it is important to continuously monitor lead integrity. It is highly desirable to discover an incipient lead problem before it results in patient symptoms or loss of treatment. Large variations in lead impedance, as well as impedances that are slowly increasing or decreasing, should always initiate an investigation and possibly also shorter follow-up intervals. This is especially true for ventricular leads and in cases where the patient is pacemaker-dependent.

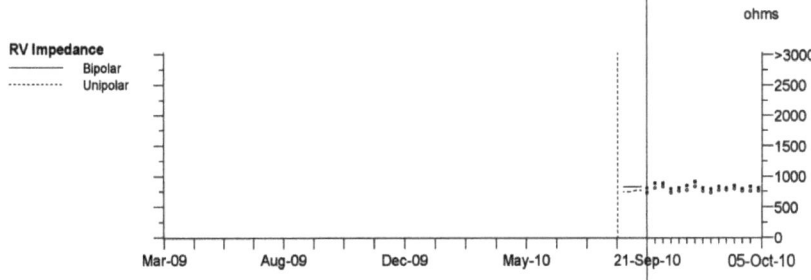

**FIGURE 8.6** Long-term ventricular impedance trend from a Medtronic EnSura

Variation in lead impedance should also prompt a comparison with other diagnostics, such as threshold and sensing trends for that particular lead. An impedance change that does not affect threshold or sensing is naturally not as grave as one that is affecting these parameters.

Early variations in impedance may be caused by so-called micro dislocation, where the lead is not yet stable against the heart wall. This will usually correct itself with time. The first impedance measurements after implant are, on some leads, quite a bit higher than the chronic values.

# The Pacemaker Battery

When developing new pacemakers, battery performance is of utmost importance. A pacemaker battery must be reliable and able to work in a hermetically closed environment, have a high energy density, and be able to provide adequate current during a long time period. The lithium battery has proven to work well, and the most common pacemaker battery today is lithium-iodine. New batteries are constantly under development, and some devices of today now use lithium/silver vanadium oxide batteries.

## Battery Measurements

Pacemaker batteries eventually discharge, and at that point the pacemaker must be replaced. When this time comes, the entire pacemaker generator is replaced; it is not possible to change just the battery. To keep track of when replacement is due, battery status is checked at each follow-up. Different manufacturers display remaining battery capacity in different ways. This can be through presenting internal battery impedance and/or battery voltage. During discharge the internal impedance of the battery will increase, which in turn leads to a decreasing battery voltage. Each particular battery has manufacturer-preprogrammed values for replacement. The pacemaker will then switch to a mode less current-draining (for example, VVI), and a message will be displayed on the programmer that the pacemaker has reached RRT (recommended replacement time). After RRT, the device generally lasts at least three more months with standard parameters, often even longer.

Many devices provide automatic calculations of the estimated remaining longevity. These calculations should not be seen as absolute values since both the battery and the pacemaker circuitry have certain tolerances that may affect the estimation. These calculations should therefore be seen more as an estimation.

When battery longevity is approaching an end, it is common to incorporate more frequent follow-ups. Different clinics have different approaches to when to replace the device. If the patient is not expected to have more than one replacement, there are no economic or medical benefits in waiting too long. It is more advantageous, both for patient and economics, to avoid frequent follow-ups, and at the same time the cost for the replacement will remain the same independently of when it is performed (given that no more replacements will be needed).

# Follow-up of the Pacemaker System

To ensure optimal treatment, the patient is called in for regular follow-up of the implanted system. This is usually done six to eight weeks after implant (the wound is also checked for any signs of infection, etc., at this time), and after that every six to twelve months. Some European clinics have even lengthened that interval to every two years in the beginning of service life, then increasing the frequency when the device gets closer to RRT.

Many devices allow for storage of patient information in the device memory. This information will then be available on each print-out, which may facilitate patient file work. Historically it was possible to follow-up a pacemaker just by applying a magnet on top of the device. This would cause the pacemaker to revert to asynchronous mode, and the pacemaker could also have some sort of threshold measurement started by magnet application. The rate with which the device was pacing (so-called magnet rate) was dependent upon battery status, and thus a battery check could be performed at the same time. Magnet function is still available with modern pacemakers, but the complexity of today's pacemakers makes it hardly possible to do a follow-up without a programmer (except for remote follow-up).

# Remote Follow-up

Remote follow-up of ICDs and pacemakers have been performed in the United States since 2002, and this was introduced in Europe some years later. In the beginning, this type of follow-up was offered mostly to ICD patients, but today pacemaker patients can also choose not to come to the hospital for routine check-ups. Instead, this can be performed from the patient's home by using a transmission monitor connected to the phone (or by a cellular SIM card) that will read and transmit data from the pacemaker to a secure server. The data is then checked by the pacemaker physician or nurse, and the patient will only have to come to the hospital if an issue needs to be addressed. This offers several advantages for the patient:

- Time saving: Working-aged patients don't need to take time off from work for follow-up, and older patients who would need help to get to the hospital don't have to have a friend or family member take a day off.
- No transportation or parking costs
- Fragile patients stressed by transportation can stay in their homes
- Children who have had a bad hospital-environment experience can be checked from home and be spared another stressful experience.

The aging population and the growing number of patients treated with a pacemaker also increases the workload in pacemaker clinics. For this reason, remote follow-up is also advantageous for the healthcare system in some ways:

- Time saving: To follow a patient remotely simply takes less time than to bring the patient into the clinic.

- Economically advantageous: Studies show that it is cost-saving to do remote follow-up when compared to in-clinic visits[4].
- Troubleshooting and interpretation of diagnostic data can be performed in a quiet environment without the patient being present, and the diagnosis and possible actions can be delivered to the patient without the worrisome experience of troubleshooting and discussions.
- Lower number of emergency visits: If the patient is reassured that everything looks fine, they are less likely to come to the hospital "just in case."
- More frequent follow-ups, such as battery checks when approaching RRT, monitoring of a suspect lead, or reading of arrhythmia diagnostics after change in medication, is more quickly performed remotely.

# Single-Chamber Follow-up

Follow-up of the single-chamber device commonly includes the following steps:
- Stimulation threshold measurement
- Sensing amplitude measurement
- Battery review and estimation of remaining longevity
- Lead impedance review
- Review of stored data and rate distribution
- Review of stored arrhythmias (if any)

---

[4] Europace. 2008 Oct;10(10):1145-51

- For unipolar sensing polarity, a muscle provocation test may be performed
- For AAI systems, a conduction test may be performed.

## The AAI Pacemaker

Follow-up of the AAI pacemaker must also include testing of the patient's intrinsic AV conduction from time to time. This should especially be the case if the patient describes symptoms (for example, during exercise). The simplest way to test AV conduction is by increasing the atrial stimulation rate to measure the Wenckebach point. The stimulation rate is increased stepwise until a Wenckebach behavior is noted on the ECG. The result is not fully reliable, however, since no stress hormones are released during such a test (hormones that would possibly shorten the PQ interval and increase the Wenckebach point). To get a more reliable result, the patient needs an exercise test where the ECG can be monitored for any AV block tendencies. If this cannot be done, it may be possible to catch the phenomenon on ECG by letting the patient exercise (walk in the corridor, climb stairs) and then monitor the ECG directly afterward, before the rate has the chance to decrease. No signs of AV block should be noted. If this is not the case, an upgrade to a dual-chamber system may be necessary.

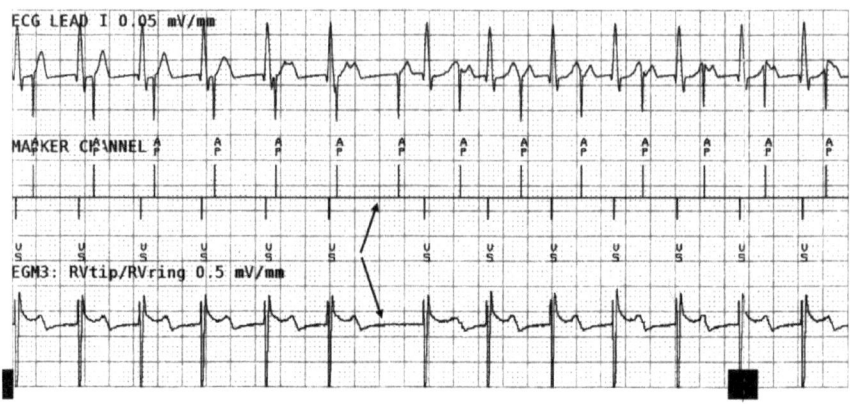

**FIGURE 10.2** AV block in AAIR stimulation during exercise. Note the prolonged conduction time and the missing (blocked) QRS marked with arrows.

## The VVI Pacemaker

VVI follow-up is slightly different from that of AAI devices. In sinus rhythm and AV block, it is not uncommon to find some degree of pacemaker syndrome since ventricular stimulation is not synchronized to the atrium. This may lead to retrograde conduction or to the atrium and ventricle contracting simultaneously. The atria will then contract against closed valves, which may cause symptoms such as dizziness, presyncope, palpitations and dyspnea. For these patients, an upgrade to a dual-chamber system may prove necessary to eliminate the symptoms. A retrograde conduction test can be performed by pacing the ventricles at different rates and looking for a correlation between ventricular stimulation pulses and (retrograde) P waves. If the P waves follow ventricular stimulation, retrograde conduction has been demonstrated. If this also leads to patient symptoms, an upgrade, as described above, may be necessary.

104

# Dual-Chamber Follow-up

Follow-up of the dual-chamber device commonly includes the following steps:

- Atrial and ventricular stimulation threshold measurements
- Atrial and ventricular sensing amplitude measurements
- Optimizing AV delay and minimizing ventricular stimulation
- Battery review and estimation of remaining longevity
- Atrial and ventricular lead impedance review
- Review of stored data and rate distribution
- Review of stored arrhythmias (if any)
- For unipolar sensing polarity, a muscle provocation test may be performed.

Follow-up of the dual-chamber pacemaker is somewhat more time consuming than that of the single-chamber device. Not only are measurements taken on two leads rather than one, but the integration of two channels (for example, AV delay) makes follow-up somewhat more complex. During dual-chamber follow-up, the working process is also more dependent upon possible ECG findings at the start of the follow-up. Do far-field signals exist? Crosstalk? Pacemaker-mediated tachycardia? To what extent is the device stimulating the ventricles? Could ventricular pacing be diminished? Is the AV delay optimal? Is there a spike-P delay? The experienced physician/nurse quickly gets an overview by studying the ECG, EGM and markers. For the less experienced, more time is needed and use of a to-do list may be helpful.

# Troubleshooting

From time to time, a system that is not working well will be discovered during follow-up. This may be found during a scheduled follow-up, or the patient may feel that something is wrong and seek help more acutely. In some cases, the patient will describe symptoms only occurring at certain instances, such as during specific activities or body movements. In those cases, it is a good idea to mimic the described situation as closely as possible to try to provoke the symptoms. With lead problems, showers of noise can often be noted on EGM and markers when the patient is doing, for example, certain arm movements, which may be possible to provoke during ECG registration.

Pacemaker generators rarely fail, while lead failures are more common. Many of those failures can be diagnosed by studying pacemaker diagnostics, ECG, EGM, markers and by performing a few simple tests. Before troubleshooting begins, it may be wise to consider whether the patient's symptoms could be related to something other than the implanted system. Perhaps comorbidity could cause dizziness, exercise intolerance, etc.?

## Strategies for Troubleshooting

Although it is not possible to give complete advice on how troubleshooting should be performed in a specific case, it is useful to have a strategy for how such a procedure could be outlined. Below is a list of suggestions that may be useful:

1. Anamnesis: When did the problem start? What symptoms are there? When do symptoms occur? Were the symptoms preceded by any special event (such as trauma, illness, change in medication, etc.)? When was the system implanted? A newly implanted system usually has different failure mechanisms than one that has been implanted longer.

2. Real time ECG with markers: Is the rhythm regular? Arrhythmias? PACs/PVCs? Undersensing? Oversensing? Exit block?
3. EGM signals: Is the amplitude varying? Are the signals smaller than expected? Far-field signals? Noise?
4. Review programming and diagnostics. Any unusual findings?
5. Depending on the nature of the problem, provocation tests may be advised. For example, it may be possible to recreate the situation that the patient describes as being symptomatic in the home environment.
6. Fluoroscopy: If lead dislodgement, lead breakage, or a poor connection in the header is suspected, fluoroscopy may add important information.

## Lead Problems

If a lead is not functioning properly, this may affect treatment in a variety of ways. A full set of diagnostic parameters may be the difference between finding the problem before it gives symptoms and a visit to the emergency room. The most commonly seen problems are listed below:

**Lead dislocation:** Most commonly seen within the first weeks after implantation. May result in exit block, undersensing, oversensing and sometimes also changes in lead impedance. It is not uncommon for a dislodged atrial lead to follow the blood stream down to the ventricle. If so, the EGM signal will help in finding where the lead is situated. As well, smaller changes in position may be found on fluoroscopy if pictures of the original position have been stored.

**Subclavian crush:** When leads are implanted using the Seldinger technique via vena subclavia, it is of great importance that the puncture is not too medial, placing the lead between the clavicle and the first rib. Leads introduced medially are exposed to higher mechanical force and have an increased risk of failing. Lead impedance trends may show decreasing impedance values (insulation failure) or increasing values (conductor break). Impedance measurements may vary, especially early on in the process (for example, with arm movements, which can be seen during repeated measurements during movements affecting the clavicular area). Large variations between values during arm movements are indications for subclavian crush, and these should prompt lead replacement of the lead. In this type of lead failure, it is common to see episodes of oversensing on the marker channel, resulting from intermittent contact between broken conductors. These episodes may also be stored in pacemaker memory as episodes of high rate. Fluoroscopy of the area around the clavicle should give information about lead placement relative to the clavicle/first rib, and conductor break or insulation failure may be visualized.

**Insulation defects:** Insulation defects may involve the outer and/or inner insulation layers. In insulation failures of unipolar leads, the current is offered a parallel shortcut to the pacemaker can through the defect. This in turn will lead to less current taking the path through the lead tip, with higher threshold and lower lead impedance as the result. Sensing also may be affected negatively. In defects on the inner insulation layer of a bipolar lead, the conductors will be short-circuited (partly or fully) and a smaller part of the current will reach the lead tip while the rest returns to the pacemaker via the short-cut. Also in this case, lead impedance decreases, threshold increases, and sensing may be affected.

**Conductor break:** Conductor break is defined as a partial or full break in the electrical conductor of the lead. The lead impedance will increase with the degree of the break, and the delivered current will decrease at the lead tip due to the increased impedance. With a full break, no current is delivered. Partial break will lead to impedance variances in conjunction with showers of noise/oversensing. Varying threshold values or exit block are common.

Lead injury may occur at different levels of the lead body, but is quite often found in or around the pacemaker pocket. Excess lead length can cause injuries due to wearing cable against cable or cable against can, resulting in insulation or conductor failure. Damage to the lead can also happen during dissection of the lead during pacemaker replacement procedures (usually insulation damage) or in the proximity of the suture sleeve used to anchor the lead in the vessel. Lead damage in the pocket is can sometimes be provoked by manipulation of the pacemaker and lead from outside of the body. This provocation should be done while closely monitoring the ECG, EGM and markers. It is very important to keep in mind that the problem *may get worse* (a partial break may turn to a complete break), which could turn out to be potentially dangerous if the patient is pacemaker-dependent.

Lead injury may also occur in locations other than the pacemaker pocket, but it will then be more difficult to provoke.

**Connector problems:** It is of utmost importance that the connection between the pacemaker and the lead is correct. The lead pin should be inserted fully into the connector, and the connector screw/screws should be carefully tightened. When fully inserted, the lead pin should be visible passed the set screw. In intermittent contact between the lead and the pacemaker, problems similar to partial cable break may be observed. Provocative testing by manipulating the lead close to the pacemaker (from outside of the body) while measuring lead impedance may show large variations and showers of oversesning. However, be aware that *intermittent contact may turn into no contact, with loss of therapy as the result*. Fluoroscopy may also reveal that the lead pin is not fully inserted. When reoperating, always attempt to pull the lead out of the connector *without* untightening the set screw first. If the lead comes out, there is proof for misconnection and other types of lead failures may be excluded. A correct reconnection of the lead should solve the problem.

# Malprogramming

As described earlier in this book, correct programming, adapted to the needs of the individual patient, is necessary to provide optimal therapy. Malprogramming can lead to a variety of symptoms, depending on what parameters need reprogramming. Some of the problems seen after malprogramming are: exit block, oversensing, undersensing, PMT, far-field sensing, pacemaker syndrome and exercise intolerance, all described in earlier chapters of this book.

# Arrhythmias

When looking for an explanation for a patient's symptoms, spontaneous arrhythmias should always be considered. These can often be diagnosed by the pacemaker diagnostics, including episodes of high rate. To achieve the desired data, it is sometimes necessary to reprogram data collection (for example, detection rates or EGM type to be stored).

# Programming
# Recommendations

**Mode**

Most commonly used is DDD/R. For patients without AV conduction disorders, AAI/R may be considered, or more commonly, modes such as Medtronic MVP to promote AV conduction. For patients with chronic atrial fibrillation/flutter, and for patients with a very sporadic need for stimulation, VVI/R is usually chosen.

**Amplitude and pulse width**

Two times safety margin from amplitude threshold, or three times safety margin from pulse width threshold is used. Values below 2 V or above 1 ms are less common, with the exception of atrial amplitude which may be programmed below 2 V when the patient is not dependent on atrial stimulation. At higher thresholds, a pulse width above 1 ms may be considered to increase safety margin without increasing the amplitude too much. Up until the first follow-up, six to eight weeks after implant, a larger safety margin is used to allow for threshold peaking.

**Sensitivity**

At least two to three times safety margin from the measured signal (i.e. the measured signal is divided by 2-3). Higher sensitivity is needed in bipolar sensing, and lower sensitivity is necessary in unipolar sensing. In the atrium, it is important to take into account whether atrial fibrillation with small amplitudes needs to be sensed. In the ventricle, PVCs and R waves may be of different sizes and call for a higher sensitivity.

**Polarity**

Bipolar sensing is less prone to oversensing of noise, but vector-dependent sensing makes the system more sensitive to undersensing. Unipolar pacing gives

| | |
|---|---|
| | pacing spikes that are clearly visible on ECG, but it may result in stimulation of the pectoral muscle. |
| **Lower rate** | Normally between 50 and 70 min$^{-1}$. In pediatric pacing, higher rates are used, adapted to the age of the child. Higher rates will shorten battery longevity. With modes allowing for rate variation, such as DDD or rate response, a lower rate may be chosen. A rate of 70 min$^{-1}$ may be tried to prevent atrial fibrillation. |
| **Hysteresis** | Mostly used in single-chamber stimulation without rate response, which is not commonly seen today. A hysteresis rate of around 10 min$^{-1}$ below lower rate, depending on the lower rate programmed, may be reasonable. |
| **Night Rate** | Is more appropriate in single-chamber stimulation. A decrease of lower rate at night with 10-20 min$^{-1}$ is helpful for some patients. |
| **Refractory and blanking** | Used in single-chamber devices. In VVI, the T wave should be covered by the blanking period if possible. In AAI, eventual far-field signals from the ventricles should be covered by blanking. For the noise reversion algorithm to work, part of the refractory period needs to be relative (i.e. not completely taken up by blanking). |
| **SAV** | Commonly 150-170 ms in AV block. Longer if intrinsic AV conduction needs to be promoted. SAV is programmed approximately 30 ms shorter than PAV if the spike-P interval is short. |
| **PAV** | Commonly 180-200 ms in AV block. Longer if intrinsic AV conduction needs to be promoted. PAV is programmed approximately 30 ms longer than SAV if the spike-P interval is short. In long spike-P intervals, the PAV is prolonged with that interval. |
| **RAAV** | Automaticity that shortens the AV interval when the heart rate is increasing. It is used in AV block III to increase the 2:1-block rate. Minimum AV should be tolerated during exercise and allow for a 2:1 block at a higher rate than the maximum rate achieved during exercise. |
| **AV hysteresis** | Switched on to promote intrinsic conduction when necessary. Adjusted to a value longer than that measured from the atrial event to the ventricular sense. |

| | |
|---|---|
| **Ventricular refractory** | Dual-chamber ventricular refractory period started in the ventricle after a ventricular event. Programmed to cover possible T waves. 230 ms is a common value. Must be shorter than PVARP. |
| **PVARP** | Dual-chamber refractory period in the atrium, started on a ventricular event. PVARP includes PVAB. PVARP should cover possible far-field signals from the ventricle and be longer than eventual retrograde conduction times from ventricular pace to atrial sense. PVARP plus SAV limits the highest atrial rate which the ventricles can follow by setting the 2:1 block rate. 2:1 block should always be avoided for rates within the patient's exercise range. Automatic shortening of PVARP at higher rates is recommended to avoid 2:1 in AV block patients. |
| **PVAB** | Blanking period in the beginning of the PVARP. To prevent far-field sensing from the ventricle from negatively affecting atrial diagnostics, and possibly causing mode-switching, it is preferable to have the PVAB covering all such signals. |
| **PMT features** | Should almost always be switched on to avoid PMT. |
| **Upper rate** | Should be kept higher than the patient's sinus rhythm during exercise to prevent symptoms. A rule of thumb could be to program UR to 220 minus patient age. Upper rate should never be higher than the 2:1 block rate. In heart failure, it is important that the patient can tolerate the programmed upper rate without symptoms. |
| **Ventricular Safety Pace** | Feature to minimize the risk of crosstalk. Should ALWAYS be enabled. |
| **Mode-switch** | Used for patients with paroxysmal atrial tachycardia to stabilize and keep the ventricular rate down. The pacemaker switches mode from DDD/R to DDI/R to turn tracking off. Mode-switch detection rate should be below the rate of the arrhythmia. The use of mode-switch for patients without known arrhythmias may be discussed. |
| **Rate stabilization during AF** | Switched on for patients with atrial fibrillation where symptoms are caused by irregularities in the rate, causing irregular filling of the ventricles. |
| **ATP therapies** | Used to stop ongoing atrial reentry tachycardia and atrial flutter. Burst or ramp protocols are tested to ensure correct function. |

**Rate response**

Sensor-driven rate to overtake the function of the sinus node to increase heart rate during exercise. Different manufacturers use different sensors and algorithms, so it is not possible to give general programming recommendations. Evaluation of the need for rate response can be done via the heart rate histogram or by performing a programmer-driven exercise test.

# References

1. Wiberg S, Lönnerholm S, Jensen SM, et al., Effect of right atrial overdrive pacing in the prevention of symptomatic paroxysmal atrial fibrillation: a multicenter randomized study, the PAF-PACE study. Pacing Clin Electrophysiol. 2003 Sep;26(9):1841-8

2. Sweeney MO., Hellkamp AS., Ellenbogen KA., et al., Adverse Effect of Ventricular Pacing on Heart Failure and Atrial Fibrillation Among Patients With Normal Baseline QRS Duration in a Clinical Trial of Pacemaker Therapy for Sinus Node Dysfunction. Circulation 2003;107;2932-2937

3. Akhtar M., Retrograde conduction in man. Pacing Clin Electrophysiol. 1981 Sep;4(5): 548–562

4. Raatikainen MJ, Uusimaa P, van Ginneken MM, et al., Remote monitoring of implantable cardioverter defibrillator patients: a safe, time-saving, and cost-effective means for follow-up. Europace. 2008 Oct;10(10):1145-51

# Index